# AGING IS INEVITABLE
# GETTING OLD IS A CHOICE

*How to Reverse Your Biological Age and
Redefine What Getting Older Looks Like*

## CARLOS CINTRON

Aging Is Inevitable, Getting Old Is a Choice: How to Reverse Your Biological Age and Redefine What Getting Older Looks Like

© 2025 Carlos Cintron



Design and cover art by Peaceful Profits.

Paperback ISBN: 978-1-967587-82-7
eBook ISBN: 978-1-967587-83-4

Hardcover: 978-1-967587-84-1

This publication is designed to provide accurate and authoritative information regarding the subject matter covered. It is sold with the understanding that the publisher is not engaged in rendering legal, accounting, or other professional services. If you require legal advice or other expert assistance, you should seek the services of a competent professional.

**Disclaimer:** The author makes no guarantees to the results you'll achieve by reading this book. All business requires risk and hard work. The results and client case studies presented in this book represent results achieved working directly with the author. Your results may vary when undertaking any new business venture or marketing strategy.

The information contained in this book is provided for educational purposes only and should not be construed as medical advice. Readers are strongly encouraged to consult with a qualified and licensed professional who can provide advice tailored to their individual circumstances. Laws, regulations, and medical practices vary across countries, states, and regions. While every effort has been made to provide accurate and timely information at the time of writing, we make no representations or warranties regarding completeness, accuracy, or applicability. We are not making any official medical recommendations. The examples, figures, and principles presented herein are for illustrative and educational purposes only. Any decisions you make are solely your responsibility.

To my father,
The Reverend Angel Luis Cintrón (1934–2025)

A man of unwavering faith, quiet strength, and boundless love. You put God first, family second, and served others with humility and grace.

You gave me life—and the values to live it with purpose. Thank you for your prayers, your example, and those birthday weights that changed everything.

This book is a tribute to your legacy and a mission we now share— helping others live with health, hope, and faith.

I love you, Pops.
Amen.


To my mother,
Maria Teresa Cintron, who passed on December 19, 2025—six months after my father.
You were my foundation, my inspiration, and my greatest teacher. Your strength, grace, and unwavering love shaped the man I've become.
Every lesson in resilience, discipline, and reinvention began with you.
This book is a reflection of your legacy—a reminder that aging is not about decline, but about how deeply one has lived and loved.
Thank you for everything you gave, and everything you were.
I carry you with me always.
I love you.
Carlos

*One of the greatest mistakes our society has made is believing that aging must come at the cost of health, strength, and vitality.*
—Carlos Cintron

# Contents

# Foreword

I t is my great privilege to introduce *Aging Is Inevitable, Getting Old Is a Choice* by Carlos Cintron. This is one of the most insightful and inspiring books ever written on health and personal well-being. You only have one body—take care of it. If you neglect it, the cost is not only physical but emotional and spiritual as well.

This book reminds us that aging is a natural process, but how we age is entirely up to us. Typically, if a book offers even one passage or idea with the power to change a person's life, that alone justifies reading it, rereading it, and finding a permanent place for it on your shelf.

This book delivers far more.

At its heart, *Aging Is Inevitable, Getting Old Is a Choice* is a story of personal development and conscious living. Carlos Cintron shares the foundations of his strength, discipline, and resilience through his framework "The 5 Elements of Life". His journey goes beyond physical fitness, it is about inner alignment, mental mastery, and the unwavering refusal to surrender to time, circumstance, or society's narrative of aging.

Carlos reminds us to never give up on life and to never lose hope for a better future. Regardless of your age, these principles apply to everyone. He believes that the best teachers are those who use themselves as bridges, helping others cross to new levels of success and inspiring them to build bridges of their own.

Through his words and example, Carlos reignites opportunities for those who may have missed them the first time or for those who wish to seize them again. In reflecting on his journey, he expresses no regrets—only determination to continue building those bridges, for himself and for all who follow.

This book is more than a guide to healthy living; it is a testament to the human spirit's capacity for growth, renewal, and purpose at any stage of life.

Written by Paul Digrigoli

Cosmetologist, entrepreneur, and author, Paul has been a mentor and lifelong friend.

# Chapter 1

# Aging in Reverse: Why This Matters Now

*The best time to plant a tree was twenty years ago.*
*The second best time is now.*
*–Chinese proverb*

I was four years old when the city bus struck me.

My mom was pushing my baby sister in a carriage through Hartford, Connecticut. I was walking alongside her, my hand in hers. Somehow, I broke away from my mother's grip and ran into the street as a bus was leaving its stop. As far as traumatic brain injuries go, I was lucky. The bus wasn't going fast—otherwise, there's no telling how my fragile skull would've fared against fifteen tons of aluminum and steel. Even so, the force fractured my skull and left contusions all over my body. I don't remember the moment of impact, only what it taught me: just how fast life can change, and how long the body keeps the ledger. It would be the first of two traumatic brain injuries

(TBIs) that shaped the way I view aging, resilience, and what it means to have a choice in how we age.

Growing up in the 1960s and 70s was the wild wild west compared to how kids grow up today. There were no conversations around health and wellness, and if there were, they were centered around the latest liquid fad diet or frozen convenience food made in the microwave like magic. When my siblings and I weren't in church, we were running around the neighborhood with our friends, grabbing whatever junk or candy we could get our hands on as kids do. We were products of our environment. I realized as I got older and became a father myself that our parents only wanted us to grow up better than they did. They didn't know what they didn't know—about health and wellness. While writing this book, I witnessed aging in its most fragile form. My father, after years of battling high blood pressure and chronic illness, suffered a devastating stroke in 2022 that left him paralyzed and ultimately led to his passing at 91. Just six months later, my 83-year-old mother—confined to a bed or wheelchair by severe osteoarthritis, high blood pressure, and dementia—followed him, a loss that profoundly shaped the message of this book.

They are my *why*. Witnessing my parents age opened my eyes and heart to the fact that we are living in a poorly aging population. *One in six people globally will be age 60 or older by 2030*—that's 1.4 billion people.[1] The problem isn't that our largest living generation is growing old, it's that we've figured out how to extend our lifespan without expanding our healthspan: the number of years we spend feeling strong, sharp, independent, and energized.[2]

I'm 62 years old, and there was a time I didn't think I'd openly admit that.

We're told that after 40 we slow down. After 50, we fade into the background. And after 60? We're lucky to be here. Honestly? That's bullshit. But stigma isn't the core problem. It's a symptom of something much more sinister: conformity.

If you take nothing else from this book, remember this: Conformity is what ages and ultimately kills you.

Replace conformity with curiosity and watch your world open up to reveal depth, meaning, and possibility beyond your wildest dreams. **Curiosity is more than a mindset shift, it's a survival skill**. A landmark study of more than 2,000 older adults found that higher levels of curiosity were directly linked to longer life, even after accounting for other risk factors.[3] Those who took a lifelong learner's mindset lived longer. Staying curious is scientifically proven to keep the aging brain and body alive and thriving. The longer I've worked in the field of regenerative medicine, the clearer it's become that aging isn't as linear as is commonly believed. The body doesn't fail us. It responds to the inputs we give it, doing the best with the information it has. Change the inputs, change the outcome. When we talk about longevity, what we're really talking about is quality of life. That doesn't come from one therapy or one supplement. It comes from living in alignment with what your body is asking for. And curiosity keeps you young.

That's why this book exists *now*. We're at a crossroads, and we're faced with a choice—to change the way we think or to stay the same.

Adults are suffering, and once your eyes are open, you can't unsee it. Western culture treats "old" like an expiration date, and you're expected to quietly step over the threshold. Dive beneath the surface into the research and you'll learn how science is rapidly developing ways to repair, restore, and protect the body and mind at every age. *And you don't hear enough about the options!* The gap between those two realities—the story you're told and the tools you have available—is the gap this book is here to close.

When I talk about aging I don't mean decline; I'm talking about change. Some of that change we can't control, sure. But we can influence an incredible amount of it. The discourse around aging centers around less: less muscle mass, less neuroplasticity, less bone density… How about we substitute old with vintage? We've never seen anyone cast aside a vintage watch or bottle of wine. There is another path—one where age can be celebrated, not hidden. This is a path where our choices compound and our bodies respond positively.

- **Lifespan** is how long you live.
- **Healthspan** is how long you live well—with mobility, clarity, purpose, independence, and most importantly, *peace.*

*So it is: We are not given a short life but we make it
short. Life is long if you know how to use it.*
*—Seneca*

For the last half century, we've focused on adding years. It's time to infuse *life* into those years. This is not theoretical; for me, it's deeply personal. I watched my father preach about hope and service, and then spend his final years in a bed trapped by a body that couldn't do what his spirit still wanted to do. I watched my mother—once a vibrant business owner and hairdresser—lose mobility and memory until her world narrowed to a few rooms. And I'm practicing, as I cross into my 60s, choosing differently. Not because I'm better, I'm a regular guy. I'm just like you. But I've learned to ask good questions; I've been curious since long before I reached middle age. Really as far back as I can remember, I've pondered my future.

Somewhere along the way your health has been outsourced to systems that are great at crisis response and not great at prevention. Who knows your body and its signals better than you? Tune in and you'll find your body already holds the answers—or at the very least, the right questions. I'm grateful for doctors; many have saved my life. But most of what determines who we become in our 60s, 70s, 80s, and beyond won't be found on an operating table or in a prescription medication. It happens in kitchens, bedrooms, parks, and gyms. In quiet morning routines and deeper spiritual practices. How well we age is a culmination of the thoughts we rehearse and habits we repeat. This book argues for a collective cognitive shift. From "this is what happens" to "what else is possible?"

## How to Use This Book

This is not a textbook nor is it a miracle-cure manifesto.

It's a field guide.

Part memoir, part map.

It's a purposely short read. I'll lay out my simple, integrated framework—The 5 Elements of Life—that I've implemented to keep my own healthspan expanding: Spirituality, Mindset, Movement, Nutrition, and Functional Medicine. You'll learn how these elements work in harmony to amplify one another, and soon implement them yourself.

The first two elements, Spirituality and Mindset, lay the groundwork, urging you to start (or strengthen, if you've already established) the same practices on which I've relied day-to-day for decades.

The third and fourth elements, Movement and Nutrition, will challenge you to look in the mirror. The person staring back can be your biggest Opponent (capital *O*; you'll soon learn why) or your greatest ally. You get to choose. I'll share why moving my body is the best part of my day and give you a guide to building movement habits for your body type and your age, decade by decade. Nutrition may feel challenging, but there's no such thing as failures, only valuable information that can guide you. The nutrition tips I share with you here have been built from decades manipulating my own body across the full spectrum—from obese to 6% bodyfat. You'll get memorable cues for portion sizes depending on your body type that you can easily recall whether you're cooking at home or away on vacation.

And finally, the fifth and most precise element is Functional Medicine. Gone are the days of guesswork. You're holding straightforward, no-nonsense therapies you can explore as soon as you flip the final page. And you'll have a fresh look at the fastest evolving science for accelerating healing and decelerating aging once your foundation is solid.

You won't find rigid rules here. I still love ice cream and enjoy a glass of wine. I have days where the lifting session feels heavier than usual and nights where my mind wants to pick at old worries. I'm not a physician; I'm a walking experiment. I've spent four decades learning my body and two decades obsessively researching how to help it heal after injury. I've made mistakes, reversed course, and found my way forward with mentors, coaches, doctors, loved ones, and a lot of trial and error. I've documented my mistakes for you so you don't have to live my journey. Instead, you can apply what I've learned to your own reality.

I'll be honest about where I've stumbled, like the season I hid my age because I was afraid of the stigma, the months I lost all sense of self, and the nights when stress made a home in my chest. I'll talk about the second traumatic brain injury that blindsided me 37 years after the first, and what both taught me about the body as a vessel. I'll share how becoming a father at 46 rewired my priorities and how a breakup at 55 finally put me in a therapist's chair. This eventually led me to find meditation, a practice that continues to change my life daily.

But I'm getting ahead of myself. The point is: I've lived the messy middle between decline and reemergence, and I know what it's like to tirelessly search for a way through.

Let's say the quiet part out loud: A lot of us are scared. Not of death, exactly, but of slow erosion. We wince at the thought of losing our edge, our role, our usefulness. We feel it when we hesitate before lifting a suitcase or forget a word mid-sentence. When we avoid the camera in group photos. When a doctor shrugs and says, "Well…that's all part of aging."

I *never* accepted that shrug!

Here's the narrative I'm inviting you to adopt:

- **Old is not an identity you have to claim.** It's a story Big Pharma sells you to grow their bottom line. You don't have to buy in.

- **Decline isn't inevitable.** Yes, wear-and-tear is real, but repair-and-restore is too. Your body is a highly intelligent regenerative miracle. Treat it like one.

- **Motivation won't help you.** Tiny consistent choices will. Ten minutes done is better than an hour paralyzed by perfectionism.

- **You're not late.** You're exactly on time to make a different next choice.

I'm not promising you'll feel 25 forever. While I take pride in looking and feeling 20 years younger than my biological age (and I have the blood panels to corroborate that statement), I'm promising that whatever age you are, you can feel more like *you* than you do right now. And when I say the body keeps a ledger, I mean everything counts. Every nourishing meal, quality night's sleep, walk in nature, and moment of laughter and connection acts as a deposit. Every chronic stressor, every time you slept only four hours, every decade you didn't move much—those are withdrawals. And it's cumulative.

Nobody's coming to save you. Nobody is going to hold your hand, motivate you, or help you face the monsters living within you. When you look the monster in the eye and befriend it, it can't hurt you anymore. In fact, maybe it can point you in the right direction. Have you ever asked it to?

You picked up this book—or perhaps were gifted it—for a reason. You too can start reversing your biological age. Anybody can! The nervous system is malleable. Muscle responds to load into our ninth and tenth decades (yes, really).[4] The brain self-cleans while you sleep.[5] The gut microbiome heals the body when you feed it what it needs.[6] Inflammation retreats when you target your inflammation markers and remove triggers.[7] Once your foundational lifestyle medicine is strong, you can call in tools: peptides, regenerative medicine, and supplements that can push aging into reverse even further. But we don't start there; we start with the base and build it 1% better daily.

## An Invitation

If you've read this far, you probably feel a tug. The thing about those tugs—maybe you call it fate, or dharma—is that we don't have the choice to ignore them forever. Much like artists or preachers, it's a vocation. The pull to take action will get stronger and stronger until you can't resist it, and hopefully not due to injury, sickness, or diagnosis. **You can change in a moment of joy and inspiration or pain and suffering.** Why wait? Love yourself enough to change before you must.

I'm not a doctor or a clinician—just someone who has spent years in the trenches of fitness, self-development, and everyday trial and error. What I share here comes from lived experience, countless conversations during my career in cosmetology, and my journey as an all-natural bodybuilder, all driven by a genuine desire to offer peer-to-peer support. Take what resonates, leave what doesn't, and always listen to your own body first.

I can't promise easy. But I can offer clarity and tools, and the rest is up to you. I can promise that if you trade conformity for curiosity, deposit more than you withdraw, and train your mind like you train your muscles, you'll feel the shift, then you'll see it. Then others around you will see it. Energy will come back online. Your mood will steady. Sleep will deepen. Joints will complain less. The mirror won't be the judge, and your waistline won't reduce your self worth to belt notches. Confidence will run deep and you'll shine from within. And when you stumble—and you will because you're human— you'll know what to do next. You'll have The Five Elements to catch you. And you'll know that your biological age is not a clock ticking down. It's a stopwatch you can reset. You're not behind. You're exactly where you're supposed to be, right on time.

00:00:00. Let's begin.

*Chapter 2*

# My Story

In the years following the bus accident, I grew into an obese child and an easy target. School was a gauntlet. Defending myself came with consequences, but fighting was the only way I knew how to quiet the noise…and the bullies. The jokes at school started as whispers and graduated to nicknames that stuck to me like burrs. I developed a thick skin and learned how to make someone laugh before they could laugh at me. Although I was broken on the inside, I always kept my sense of humor and my friends on the outside of an impenetrable exterior.

Thoughts could turn dark in a heartbeat. When you're a preteen trying to make sense of the world, carrying around insecurity, you're already bearing enough weight. I was tired of being fat and of the constant comparisons my brain would make between me and my brother and me and my friends who seemed more at ease in their skin. The voices that belonged to my low self-esteem would get louder around people. Feeling most alone surrounded by people who care about you…that's its own kind of loneliness.

My brother was the first person to make happiness feel possible. Four years my senior, he was everything I wasn't: confident, fast, athletic, the kind of dude every girl wanted to date and every guy wanted to be. He was also my greatest ally and never pitied me. When I was 10 he suggested I go out for our youth football league, convincing me my size could be an advantage, he'd say, "That's exactly what tackles and guards are for!"

For the first time, I let myself believe I could be more than just the fat kid.

The tryout wasn't the hard part. The hard part came after I'd made the team. My brother was elated, and despite being the fattest kid on the field, I was pretty happy too. The locker room, though, was a different story. I'd walked in to collect my uniform and could tell by the coach's face something was wrong. He disappeared into the back and returned a couple of minutes later, handing me the biggest jersey he could find.

It didn't fit.

There's a particular silence that settles when no one knows where to cast their eyes. I carried that silence home like yet another weight too heavy for a kid my age. I didn't play that season. I shut down, pretended I didn't care. I cared. But I went back to exactly how I'd been living before tryouts. Depressed, anxious, and emotionally eating. Then, as a freshman in high school, something new happened—girls.

For my fifteenth birthday I'd asked my father for a set of sandweights. They were all the rage in 1977! The set came with a bench, 110 pounds of weights, and a stapled booklet with black-and-white diagrams for each muscle group. There were no distractions before internet and cell phones, so I got to it. Working out became my first reliable promise to myself. I soon became obsessed. My friends would come over to train and when they went home I'd go for jogs around the block.

The weights began to feel lighter. The weight on my chest did too.

Within six months I could feel my body obeying new orders. I'd lost 50 pounds and had become unrecognizable. That was the first time I learned how small choices compound. What I didn't know back when my father gave me those weights was how I was creating new neural pathways in my brain, which sent signals to my body. I had a purpose—the drive to improve my physique and quiet the inner noise—albeit, only to get a girlfriend at first.

The summer before sophomore year, I committed myself to getting fit. I'd wanted to go out for the football team the coming fall so I was either in the gym or running, always working out like crazy. By the time school started and tryouts rolled around I had gotten myself into amazing shape.

My brother had graduated the spring prior, and I finally felt free to come into my own identity as Carlos instead of his fat younger brother. I blossomed. The football coaches were equally as impressed with the progress I had made during the summer break and my performance during two-a-day practices. I made the varsity team. The glory was short-lived though, and I'll never forget how it felt when my football dreams came crashing down. The coaches were talking about what position I was going to play for a huge game coming up. I was feeling GREAT…until I got called into the coach's office the day before our first game. He said he had some bad news and that he tried everything to get it straightened out, but unfortunately I wasn't eligible to play football because of my grades.

For a 15-year-old, that was crushing.

Coach told me if I got my grades up I'd probably be able to play after the first semester, but I was so mad I shut down the whole idea. I still worked out, just not as part of the football team. I continued going through the motions and teen life evened out—not Hollywood-movie perfect—but survivable and sometimes sweet. I dated my high school sweetheart into our 20s, and we would later marry and divorce. (I'm blessed she's still in my life as a good friend to this day.)

Reflecting back now, I wasn't aware as a kid that some of the choices I made and emotions I felt were because of my injuries at four years old.

The unrest in my brain never fully quieted. I didn't think of it as ADHD or connect it to the TBI back then; I just assumed school wasn't for me. Socially, I kept up appearances. My sense of humor was a disguise for the darkness of my innermost thoughts. I rebelled, wanting nothing to do with football after getting kicked off the team for my grades. I did end up returning to football but not until my junior year. Academically,

I faltered. Classrooms felt like cages, lectures like static. I did what was required to pass but never felt like any of it mattered. School never clicked. Unlike the gym, where everything had a formula: 10 reps. Short rest. 10 more reps. Repeat. Working out gave me a sense of accomplishment and a kind of control over my brain and body I wasn't fully aware was lacking in other parts of my life at that point. In the gym, I entered a flow state.

I finished high school knowing I wasn't headed to college. And while every young athlete dreams of playing in the league, I knew I wasn't good enough to get drafted. I wasn't going to follow my brother into the military mostly because I had a long ponytail that I didn't want to cut off, which is even funnier now that I'm bald. I needed to earn money somehow, so I took a 9-to-5 with the state of Connecticut as a storekeeper. It came with a steady paycheck, and I lasted as long as you can last in a job you hate before you start looking for exits around every corner.

The gym stayed my second home. One afternoon as I was lifting weights by myself, a guy approached and asked if I was a bodybuilder. I balked—*me?* He said I had the physique if I wanted to train for it. For whatever reason, imposter syndrome probably, I didn't say yes that day. But on the way home I ducked into a magazine shop and picked up every piece of bodybuilding literature I could find in the magazines: *Flex, Muscle & Fitness*, and *Muscular Development*. I studied them like holy texts, conquering the demons that plagued my childhood one sweaty, exhausting, demanding gym session at a time.

A year later I decided to enter my first show, the National Physiques Committee New England Championships in Hartford. When I arrived at the show, I remember feeling the self-doubt creeping in. I guess I hadn't truly mastered those voices from my childhood; I'd just muffled them under muscles and an ego every 20-something armors themselves with. All I could do was keep reminding myself to *just have fun, you got this.* I was slotted to compete in the Novice Category with eight other men. Nerves really ramped up backstage and I was acutely aware I didn't *really* know what I was doing. I could tell that the majority, if not all, were on steroids, and I knew I stood no chance against their size as a natural competitor. I didn't let that stop me from getting on stage, doing my best to copy the basic posing moves I'd learned from the magazines I'd been studying. I pushed past self-doubt, went out there, and gave each pose my best effort. Under the lights, the nerves disappeared, and my confidence skyrocketed. It felt like it all happened in a blur and, despite my lack of stage experience, I had a blast! Though I didn't place, I walked off that stage with something better than a trophy: self-validation. I'd pushed through fear of failure and followed through on something I'd set my mind and heart toward. I wanted more of that feeling— that sense of confidence and accomplishment from within. How far could this go if I kept learning how to build my body? I met a couple of the other bodybuilders backstage and got pointers on what I needed to do to prepare better the next time. To my surprise, it all had to do with nutrition.

One of the more experienced competitors suggested I check out Arnold Schwarzenegger's *Encyclopedia of Modern*

*Bodybuilding*. It changed my life. Within those pages I learned you can build your body the way architects build houses: plan the blueprint, lay the foundation, put in the work, fine-tune systems. Discipline and consistency over motivation. Purpose over ego. When it came to my training, I wasn't chasing first place as much as I was sculpting new versions of my own identity.

Meanwhile the 9-to-5 gnawed at me. My mother, who I'd witnessed build a successful business as a cosmetologist growing up, said, "You should go to cosmetology school."

"Mom, you're joking right?" I guess I stereotyped men in that field. The first thought that came into my head was *What are my friends going to think of me?*

I love and respect my mother and saw how successful she was—a celebrity hairdresser on TV back then. She was the breadwinner in our household.

"Just go to the orientation. See if you like it," she told me.

So I went, and I did like it. It was a choice that would later give me a rockstar career as not only a celebrity hairdresser, but as an award-winning creative director for an international brand. It allowed me to travel the world and work with top designers at fashion weeks in New York, Milan, and London. In 2011, I won the Texture Category at the North American Hairdressing Awards (NAHA) and was runner-up for North American Hairdresser of the Year.

But if you had told me any of that during orientation I wouldn't have believed you! I was one of two men in a room of women.

It should have felt like a dare, but it felt like oxygen. Doing hair wasn't about vanity; it was about transformation. It was about listening. I was helping people feel like the best version of themselves. Confidence shines from within. I followed in my mother's footsteps, and the practical skills came easily, probably from years of osmosis. I impressed my teachers with how effortlessly I maneuvered my tools.

After graduating cosmetology school I worked my way from mom's assistant to owning my own salon. I then transitioned out of my successful business to head the Toni&Guy flagship salon (later TIGI Bed Head) on 61st and Madison in New York City right across from Barney's. I went from clients who told me about their dog and grandkids to clients who flew in before late-night talk shows. I met celebrities, quickly went through two passports, demonstrated on huge hair stages, won awards, and even attended Vidal Sassoon's 70th birthday party in London.

Some people drink when they're overwhelmed. I get curious. If something feels confusing or scary, I seek solid ground in research and statistics. As my life and career got busier and the pressure got tougher, that's exactly what I did. And that's how Tony Robbins entered my world.

A friend and a mentor of mine, Paul Digrigoli, first introduced me to Tony's work. Paul was five years my senior with a successful cosmetology career and two salons, and he was into personal development. He was a phenomenal public speaker, so I followed suit. I took a public speaking course at Dale Carnegie, and the skills I gained proved indispensable for my career and my life. Seeing how successful Paul was, I absorbed anything he recommended like a sponge. His recommendation: *Awaken The Giant Within* by Tony Robbins. I began to take a deeper dive into my own personal development by way of Tony. His early tapes (yes, tapes) cut straight through my fog. *Change your state, change your story,* Tony exhorted. When I heard him put it that way, my world began to make sense. I was in control. It was my mind creating my reality and all its shortcomings. I started to see my mind as a powerful tool for the first time—more powerful than I knew then.

Two weeks after reading *Awaken The Giant Within*, I spotted a new client appointment in my book: Anthony Robbins. Call it fate or a date with destiny, it was a moment that changed my life and mindset forever. They say don't meet your heroes for fear it'll shatter the facade. But I met Tony Robbins in a hair chair, not an arena. He became my client. We talked while I worked and it felt like a free hour of life coaching. The guy you hear on stage—the larger than life personality with a million dollar smile—that guy lives in quiet rooms too. He always took time to ask me what was going on in my life, in my work, and what my goals were. He'd kind of challenge me in those conversations, keeping me on my toes. We became friendly, but I was cognizant of not taking advantage of his time and interest in my personal development. I constantly strived to do better, and those conversations with Tony accelerated my role within the company because I learned to become a leader. I still keep *Awaken the Giant Within* on my desk to this day.

After eleven years in the cosmetology business and with five body building shows under my belt, I relocated to Dallas with my wife at the time. That's when I really learned about what it took to be a highly competitive bodybuilder. One day during my workout at a gym called Natural Bodies, I was approached by this big muscular guy named Brian Crull, aka Mr. America *and* Mr. USA. We hit it off. After I shared my whole story with him, Brian saw my potential and asked me to join his bodybuilding team—a hand-selected group he personally trained and prepared for the most coveted shows in Texas. Those shows were held by the same bodybuilding organizations where the guys in the magazines I read as an ambitious teen had competed. We were soon mapping out my next two shows, Southwest Natural and Heart of Texas. I made it on the podium in both and I competed in two more shows with Brian as my coach. I went all natural—up against 'roiders who had been on magazine covers and in the sport way longer than I had been.

My two most honorable moments both happened in 1998. Fresh after winning his first of eight Mr. Olympia titles, Ronnie Coleman came on as guest poser at the Heart Of Texas and wouldn't you know, he was the one who handed me my second-place trophy. Then Dorian Yates, six-time Mr. Olympia, was a guest poser at the Southwest Natural where, again, I placed second and received my trophy from him. This type of achievement was beyond my wildest dreams—from an obese kid to a competitive natural bodybuilder at the highest level.

In 2002, at the peak of my cosmetology career and bodybuilding pursuits, came the second blow.

I was on stage in Vietnam at a hair show. Lights on, mic hot, adrenaline pumping the way it does when you perform for an audience. Accidents don't check the schedule. One moment I was in my element; the next, the world tipped. An opera pit rig that never made it back up to stage level. A step backwards and I fell—12 feet down. My head met hard floor, unconscious. Nose broken. Two tendons in my shoulder torn from the impact. I was wheeled into an ambulance, and on the ride from the event to the hospital my head was spinning. *I'm scared,* thoughts reeling, *How am I going to get the medical attention I need in a third world country? I need to get home NOW.* Among all the chaos, as I was pulled from the ambulance, I heard someone speaking English…was I imagining it?

I wasn't. A doctor from Los Angeles was in Vietnam training doctors and, by the grace of God, took care of me. They had only an X-ray machine, which couldn't see the extent of the damage to my shoulder. I needed an MRI. All I could think about was getting back home as soon as possible. The doctor told me he couldn't let me fly because I had a concussion, but if I came back to see him again the following day he would be able to clear me.

I went to see him the next day and was cleared to fly back to America, where I saw my doctor as soon as I could. He gave me the MRI and career-killing news: I'd be in a sling for six months. He told me if I were a professional baseball player he'd be saying I'd never play another game, as two tendons in my shoulder were basically gone, but I was determined to get back to my cosmetology career in any capacity. My doctor would also say the words I already knew in my gut: *traumatic brain injury.*

The first taught me how fast life can change. The second TBI taught me how, despite being at the height of my career and in competitive physical shape for an extreme sport, I'm not bulletproof. This was a turning point, a moment in my life where things were about to dramatically change and not from a moment of joy and inspiration, but because of pain and suffering.

*Chapter 3*

# The 5 Elements of Life!

*The greatest medicine of all is to teach
people how not to need it.
–Hippocrates*

Recovery is boring on purpose. It's not a montage like in the movies. It's frustration and medication and short walks and saying no to things you used to say yes to. If you're paying attention though, recovery humbles you into recognizing the divine intervention in redirection.

I remember the fog in the months that followed the accident: headaches that hummed like bad wiring, my memory like a filing cabinet scattered across the floor. I'm not proud of this, but it's reality for many, myself included. Prescription hydrocodone led to the scary and helpless sort of painkiller addiction that so many recovering from injuries are unwittingly driven to. Without the pills, that searing pain in my shoulder would return. Anger and irritability took up residence in a house that used to be patient. The bodybuilder with the megawatt smile posing on stage felt so far from who I was. I was unraveling.

My career as an award-winning hairdresser was never the same after the injuries to my shoulder. I couldn't hold a blowdryer up for any extended length of time. Thank God for my accolades, because I was able to pivot into a general manager role. In 2011, I became the first vice president of education for Morracanoil, but none of it felt like I was in my element anymore. If you've ever outgrown something you love, you know how grief and relief can arrive in the same instant. I felt guilty about the relief that came from moving in a new direction, but I also knew I'd squeezed every bit out of my chapter in cosmetology. I could feel it was time for change, but this time was different. I felt hopeful—the shift spurring from a place of joy and inspiration—and went on to discover my new purpose at age 50. I was able to trust in God that He was redirecting me somewhere I was meant to be.

If there's a pattern to my life, it's this: Every challenge presents a door I didn't know I needed to open. The hinge is almost always curiosity. That curiosity after my second TBI is what eventually led me to look at health as something bigger than bodybuilding training or recovering from my injuries.

What I learned through my recovery and throughout my life is true wellness isn't found in a single habit or product. It's a system built on five interconnected elements. Each one supports the others, forming the foundation for healthspan *and* lifespan. These five elements are the fuel that power life as a whole person experience.

**Spirituality**: Your connection to something greater than yourself drives your purpose.

**Mindset**: How you think, speak, and feel about aging affects how you age.

**Movement**: You don't stop moving because you age. You age because you stop moving.

**Nutrition**: What you eat is more than fuel; it's an instruction manual for your cells.

**Functional Medicine**: Regenerative medicine and supplementation *is* preventative medicine.

Mind-body-spirit integration is the foundation of living younger, longer.

Traditional Western medicine teaches solutions to symptoms, often using medications that create new ones in the process. We live in a system that treats symptoms instead of addressing causes.

A pill for an ill.

A drug for your pain.

A prescription for sleep.

Another for the side effects.

It's not that medicine doesn't save lives; it does. *But dependence has replaced prevention.*

The data is clear:

More than **27 million Americans live with autoimmune diseases**—a group of over 100 conditions where the body's immune system mistakes its own healthy tissue for foreign invaders and it attacks itself. Women account for 80% of those affected in the US. On a global scale, approximately 10% of people—or 700 million to 800 million people worldwide—are living with at least one type of autoimmune disorder. Autoimmune diseases are more common than thought in years past and are expected to continue rising in prevalence.[8]

**Mental health disorders have risen almost 50% since 2022**, impacting 970 million people worldwide. Anxiety is now the most common mental health issue affecting 284 million people.[9]

In the 2023–2024 academic year, 22% of college students reported taking an antidepressant the previous year. In 2007, it was 8%.[10]

**Cardiovascular disease (CVD) rates are up 4% since 2022.** This was the first increase in several years. The reversal in progress means the US is experiencing a near decade of lost progress in reducing CVD mortality with a significant number of excess deaths occurring since 2020. Contributing factors include rising rates of obesity and diabetes, which are major drivers of heart conditions.[11]

And according to the American Cancer Society, while *cancer deaths are decreasing, new diagnoses reached over 2 million* in the US in 2023, an increase from the year before.[12]

**We're living longer but not better.** Our healthcare model is excellent at emergency intervention and poor at long-term prevention. Genetics account for part of the story, but lifestyle and environment drive the majority of chronic disease. This is the basis of *epigenetics*—the science showing that our behaviors and environment influence how our genes express themselves. Nutrition, exercise, stress, sleep, and even mindset all send molecular signals that can turn genes on or off.[13]

That means our destiny is not locked in by our biology. You have control over how your body ages and adapts. Medication has its place, sure, but it's not the only answer. The foundation of health is built on daily choices. The earlier you take ownership of those choices, the more power you have to change the trajectory of your health.

Integrated practices like traditional Chinese medicine (TCM) and functional medicine (FM) examine symptoms as signals or indicators of deeper imbalances, and aim to treat the root cause through multiple healing modalities. When we only treat the surface, we merely survive. When we treat the root, we can begin to heal from the inside out.

## What actually causes the body to age?

The notion that we die of old age is one of modern medicine's most misleading myths. We do not die of old age, but of cumulative system failures inside the body. These breakdowns are not inevitable—they're reversible. Poor nutrition, lack of movement, unrelenting stress, draining relationships, and insufficient sleep fuel *inflammaging*: chronic low-grade inflammation and oxidative stress. Inflammaging underlies most of what's dismissed as "normal aging," like cardiovascular disease, type 2 diabetes, arthritis, Alzheimer's disease, sarcopenia (loss of muscle mass), even certain cancers.[14]

Inflammation is a precursor, like the emergency floor lights on an aircraft that guide you towards safety in the event of a power outage. Treating inflammation alone won't get you there. Follow the inflammation to find and heal the root cause.

---

It's funny now to think about the two instances in life that caused me to start lying about my age. At 16 I used to lie and say I was 18 to get into night clubs. In my 40s I started lying again, when younger women were drawn to me because I was physically attractive and always had a youthful aura. In 2009, my daughter Sophia was born. I was 46. If you want a masterclass in confronting time, have a kid later in life. I wanted to be the dad who could play on the floor, who could carry her when she fell asleep in the car seat. I didn't lie because I felt old, but because I didn't want to be perceived that way. As she got older I saw how proud she was to have a dad who looked and acted more youthful than other parents. That's when it hit me—why was I still hiding my age?

You can shrink from it. Or you can decide to embrace it. Being an older father taught me to move to the beat of a different drum. When I turned 50, I finally said to myself: *Carlos, you are a gift, so use your youthful aura, vitality, physicality as your super power!* That mindset shift made me a magnet, as authenticity will do to a person. There's a positive development that comes with age—embracing your own skin and stepping into your authenticity. The stigma that comes from society about aging, that's the lie. Not long after I began celebrating my true self, I began witnessing other parents, especially the dads, become more inspired to own their health no matter their ages. They would ask me questions about my routine and what my "secret" was. Now I get to reclaim my youth from within with preventative and regenerative medicine. We'll get into that in the coming pages.

**Internal wellness creates external beauty**. I wasn't chasing my youth any longer. I was choosing to stay capable for reasons bigger than myself—for those I loved. Sophia didn't just make me a father, she made me accountable to the future I kept saying I wanted.

Years later I went through a breakup that rocked my world. I felt like I lost my identity. And it felt like I lost the one person who could turn down the noise in my head to allow me to hear my own voice again. The volume came back and the voice turned self-loathing and apathetic, ruminating daily about the what-ifs. I'd hit my rock bottom—the lowest I've ever been.

I didn't know what else to do, so I walked myself into therapy and told the truth. The consultation session didn't give me answers so much as it handed me better questions. But I was skeptical at first. My therapist wasn't a traditional clinician. He believed in mind, body, and spirit.

"Learn to quiet your mind. Disease comes from dis-ease," he said. I wasn't buying the whole woo-woo meditation thing because in the same breath he also told me my chakras were out of alignment. *I'm paying this guy to help ease my pain and suffering and he's telling me I need to meditate and that my chakras are crooked?* I wanted the quick fix. But as unfamiliar as I was with the concept, I appreciated his straightforwardness in sharing this perspective: My suffering was based in my thinking and if I wanted to get through this, if I wanted to overcome my fears and feelings, it was 100% up to me. Fear exists only in the mind. That conversation was the first time I realized mindset is medicine.

Let me tell you something. The silent destroyer of self-esteem is your mind. My old mental wounds stem from being an overweight kid, and the effects have the potential to far outlast those of any physical injury. You hold more power than you think you do; you can change the trajectory of your whole life with your mind simply by noticing your inner self-talk. I do this every morning when I pray, set intentions, and meditate. Practicing mindset daily adds up to a lifetime of change. For me, those changes manifest as a sense of calm, positivity, love, and clarity.

I fell into regenerative medicine almost by accident. Call it divine intervention; call it coincidence. Whatever you attribute it to, I like to think I found my calling from walking in alignment with my purpose and being in the right place at the right time. One day in 2018, months after starting my therapy journey, a buddy called me up and said, "You should come to this regenerative medicine conference with me." I said yes immediately. I still had nagging pains and inflammation in my body from my prior injuries. Maybe something I learned here would help. We walked into the convention hall where everything that felt scattered within me would start to line up.

Little did I know I was walking into one of the largest regenerative medicine summits in the world! I had no plans to reinvent my career in biotech (although that's eventually what happened). I went because I was on a quest to discover places I could exist that weren't in my own head.

In the first lecture the speaker started talking about stem cells and I felt something click into place. I remember thinking, *Why don't more people utilize this?* He described mesenchymal stem cell (MSC) exosomes—the tiny messengers that our cells use to signal repair, and why the body loses its ability to recover as it gets older. MSC exosomes play a role in cell-free therapy, treating many diseases like cancer and aging, and are known to regulate the fate of a tumor cell.[15]

If you've lived with brain fog for any period of time, you don't need diagrams to tell you something's broken. But when I saw a presentation on neurodegenerative diseases and TBI was one of the slides, I got so emotional I felt my eyes well with tears of joy. I was looking at my struggles blown up on a projector screen and finally felt validated for what I had only known as my own experience. When I learned that MSC exosomes can cross the blood-brain barrier, I realized I could be looking at a solution to optimize my brain post-traumatic injury.

The *ah-ha!* moment was followed by questions. I was excited and intrigued, my thoughts firing off like little electrical storms over the dark city grid that was my brain. *Could this help more people with injuries like mine? What about everything else we blame on "just getting older"? Why do we treat symptoms with prescriptions without addressing the root cause?* I sought out functional medicine doctors in attendance and had illuminating conversations. I asked questions. I listened twice as much as I spoke. I left the summit with a handful of business cards and a feeling I hadn't had since I was a teenager with some sand weights and the *Encyclopedia of Bodybuilding*.

Here's the key that life handed me and functional medicine turned: The choices you make daily—how you move, eat, rest, and think—are like soil conditions of your life. Regenerative therapies are like seeds you plant in that soil. Bad soil doesn't make a bad seed; it makes growth unlikely. Conversely, good soil doesn't guarantee a harvest, it only makes one possible. You cannot out-regenerate a bad lifestyle any more than you can fix a bad golf swing with a new club. Get your reps in. The results will follow.

That summit didn't save me, but it gave me language and direction. Once again, I found solace in the research. I read about the science of regenerative medicine and learned about stem cells, MSC exosomes, and cell-based therapies. I learned the difference between what's promising in the field and what's proven. As a new representative for a reputable biotech lab, I experienced how much people want simple and honest answers in a field that often overpromises and undertranslates. I'd already spent decades learning how to be a good communicator in salons and on stages. That skill suddenly had a new assignment.

My story isn't your story. I offer it because we live inside narratives we didn't choose: *You're too old to start. You missed your window. This is just how people get at your age.* It's not my job to argue with your beliefs. It's my job to show you what happened when I argued with mine and what became possible when I replaced them.

Being an older father taught me patience and love. Training my body out of obesity taught me self-belief and perseverance. Two TBIs taught me not to take life for granted. Cosmetology taught me how to communicate and connect; bodybuilding taught me self-discipline and confidence; Tony Robbins taught me how we are more powerful than we know. My parents taught me morals, values, and trust in God. My daughter Sophia taught me why all of it matters.

Why should you care? Because getting older is a magnificent adventure you can experience on your own terms and with intention. You don't need to copy my steps. You need to choose yours. The rest of this book will show you how.

How can we prove it? We'll discuss the numerous studies on how beliefs about aging affect lifespan and healthspan. We'll talk about laying an unshakable base through spirituality and mindset—two overlooked components to aging healthfully. We'll examine how regenerative therapies team up with movement and nutrition to build a functional health picture for someone in their 60s through their 90s and even into their 100s! Above all, we'll build a framework to live daily—The 5 Elements of Life.

For now, know this: The narrative around aging is changing. You can be part of the collective shift.

# Chapter 4

# Spirituality

*You are not a human being having a spiritual*
*experience. You are a spiritual being*
*having a human experience.*
*–Pierre Teilhard de Chardin*

When you hear the word spirituality you might shy away from it or brush it off as abstract and mystical. But hear me out—spirituality lives in the body. It's not a foo-foo cloud you drift through. Spirituality is a state you cultivate through connection, calm, and consistently revisiting how it looks in practice for *you*.

When you practice gratitude, pray, meditate, or simply take a quiet walk outside, your body shifts gears from fight-or-flight to rest-and-repair. That shift is physiological. The parasympathetic nervous system activates to downshift your heart rate, your cortisol levels drop, inflammation calms, and your body finally has a chance to heal. When you feel safe, your cells feel safe. Only then does mental clarity improve, hormones balance, and recovery actually stick. Science confirms what the spiritual practices have always known: peace is medicine.[16] And it's through spirituality—whatever yours looks like—that peace and purpose can reveal themselves. For me, spirituality and its connection to a fulfilled life was modeled long before I understood it, in the quiet faith of my father.

A reverend and social worker, my father was a very spiritual and religious man. It was his vocation, I believe, because he was even named Angel. As a kid I was in church three days a week and twice on Sundays for many years. I'd longed to trade pews for bike rides with friends and spent sermons daydreaming about the Cowboys game and whoever they were facing that week. My father did a lot of things that I didn't understand growing up, like missionary trips in Haiti, Dominican Republic, and Mexico. It was evident as kids that to him God came first, and family second. While I always believed in God, I resisted religion as a kid because it felt like I had no choice in the matter. And I became resentful, I think, because I just wanted to be with my friends. It felt like I was missing out on a lot, and I didn't have much else happening in my life that brought me joy those years due to the low self-esteem. I connected the idea of church with robbing me of time just being a kid. My father was very strict. By the time I was around 17 I'd made up my mind, telling him "I'm not going." Turns out, he was also right about a thing or two, and spirituality has since returned, acting as an anchor for my faith, beliefs, and purpose through good times and bad.

My relationship with God took on different looks over the decades, and at times it had no active place in my life at all, until

I discovered Kabbalah in early 2025. Kabbalah is the ancient spiritual science of energy and consciousness. It's like a map that asks and explains everything you feel, but can't see—the soul, the connection between cause and effect, the structure of the universe in all realms of existence. It's more a framework of beliefs that underlies all faiths, philosophies, and sciences than a religion. Over the years I've learned what iteration of spirituality fills my own cup from an open and curious place, a complete 180 to how I'd experienced faith and spirituality as a kid. It stopped looking like church attendance and started taking on characteristics like gratitude, breath, and service. **Spirituality doesn't lean on any religion. It is the alignment of your thoughts, words, and actions**. And when you're living in alignment, a clear sense of purpose becomes the byproduct. Your purpose is crafted singularly for your unique gifts. Purpose is like a conductor directing all your magic—that inner alignment—outward into the real world.

Kabbalah teaches that life is not random. What's meant for you cannot miss you. Every event, every encounter, and every emotion is a coded message from the Creator guiding the soul toward transformation. In this view, the Creator is not a being, but an infinite field of light that embodies wisdom, love, compassion, and unity. An energy. A law in physics called the conservation of energy states that energy cannot be created or destroyed, only transferred and transformed.

God, Creator, Spirit, Source, Universe—call it whatever feels right. I like to say, believe in a higher power, as long as it ain't you.

## Why Spirituality Becomes Crucial as We Age

As we grow older and become more aware of mortality, the illusion of physical permanence begins to fade. **The body weakens, but the soul yearns for meaning**—remembrance of why it came into this life. Spirituality gives us meaning and that meaning, our purpose, is the visible result of the invisible inner work. It reminds us not to normalize something just because it's common, like feeling uncomfortable in our bodies, feeling lethargic, feeling tired or disconnected. Instead it urges us to treat ourselves with compassion because we're here for a reason…one no other being on the planet can replicate. It drives us out of bed when motivation dwindles (as it always will, because nothing lasting is built on motivation). Kabbalah teaches that aging and death are not punishments at all, but transitions of consciousness. Exploring spirituality helps us release fear—of failure, success, or being seen trying—and embrace purpose. Aging becomes a process of evolution, not decline. And mortality becomes a teacher of humility and gratitude; it instills a renewed urgency to live into our light fully.

Without a pursuit for spiritual understanding, life seems random and suffering meaningless. Your *why* turns into *why me?* because it's not anchored to a sound foundation—one of hope and purpose. With spirituality, every challenge becomes part of the very reason for your soul's incarnation.

You'll feel the glimmers when you're on the path to what you were put here to do. The universe starts winking at you through signs or synchronicities or coincidences that simply can't be ignored. Can you think of a time you experienced a synchronicity that you might not have noticed in the moment? I can. Seeing the name Anthony Robbins in my appointment book just two weeks after reading *Awaken The Giant Within* was a wink from the universe. Getting invited to the regenerative medicine summit and attending on a whim—another wink. God was whispering to me in those moments, urging me along a path meant only for me.

---

I've mentioned motivation a few times in this book. Let's debunk this idea as we know it and instead find its connection to spirituality. All aspects of a balanced life—mindset, movement, nutrition, and functional medicine—operate in the physical dimension. Spirituality governs the energetic and causal dimension that precedes all others. Every imbalance, whether emotional, physical, or mental, begins as a disconnection from our light. When we align our consciousness with divine energy through intention, gratitude, and awareness, we invite harmony into every area of our lives. The Kabbalists say where there is light, darkness cannot dwell.

In the context of Kabbalah, the human being is a dual system: It is ego—the desire to receive for the self alone, and soul—the desire to share. The ego seeks pleasure, control, and validation; the soul seeks purpose and light.

**Discipline, not motivation, is the path away from the confines of ego and into the freedom of the soul.** Sounds backwards, I know. But within your disciplinary habits is an alignment between your thoughts and actions, keeping promises to yourself and following through on what you said you were going to do. You're empowering yourself to grow and make choices that are in alignment with your purpose or your light. For example, staying disciplined with a diet and exercise routine gives you the freedom to feel your best and be fully present to connect with others during social events without the negative vibrations of guilt and shame hanging over you. That's living in your light! And here's where spirituality really ties in—discipline loves a *why*. Discipline underlines what you'll learn in the coming chapters on movement and nutrition, so hold on to this thought.

If you haven't already, think about your *why*. Write it down. Putting pen to paper is a powerful practice in manifestation. If manifesting is too woo-woo for you, think about it this way. Handwriting your *why* somewhere you can see often, like on your fridge or setting a photo of it as your phone background will keep you on course. Without spirituality and without your *why*, even success feels hollow. **The ego yearns for comfort; the soul yearns for growth.**

It's direction, not drive, that dwindles as people age. Aging adults stop seeing themselves as part of something bigger and start living on autopilot, giving into a stigma society holds around aging. Days blur into months and years, goals shrink, and before long you're surviving, not living.

Spirituality interrupts that drift. It's here to remind you that your existence matters and even the most mundane moments can feel extraordinary when they're connected to meaning. Have you ever watched a sunrise? There's nothing more mundane than the rotation of the earth, causing the sun to rise in the east every 24 hours—it's been happening that way since the dawn of time. Yet when you're sitting on a coastline watching that little orb of light grow bigger over the water, painting the sky above in a mosaic of pinks and oranges, it feels like it's happening just for you.

If you rest but never feel rested, eat but never feel satisfied, and find yourself reaching for distractions on your phone, convincing yourself that that's "just the way you are," **the habits you believe are protecting you are only preventing you from growth.** That's not lack of willpower, but lack of faith. People, throughout life, start to experience more anxiety as they grow older. In my experience, they haven't made peace with mortality. When we foster faith in something beyond what we can see, it helps us feel more at peace with the unknown.

What feels scarier—navigating change or living the rest of your years exactly the same? You can teach an old dog new tricks. Call on your *why* to remind you why you started.

## Trust and Certainty Beyond Logic

To trust in the light—your light—even when logic, science, or circumstance can't explain the outcome, is a state of consciousness, not naive faith. It is **spiritual intelligence**. Knowing everything that happens, even pain, has a divine architecture designed for our soul's growth is the bridge between apathy and transformation. When facing illness, crisis, or loss, our reactive nature (in Kabbalah, our Opponent within) feeds doubt, fear, and despair. The moment we acknowledge that inner Opponent and instead choose certainty—not because we can see the outcome, but because we *know* there's a greater purpose at play—we reconnect to the Creator's energetic field and true miracles are given opportunity to occur. Where there is certainty, there is light. This certainty doesn't deny pain; it transcends pain. It invites the soul to lead rather than the ego to react. It's the practice of thinking *This is hard, and I don't understand it yet, but I trust that there is light in this darkness, and I am certain I can keep going.*

Certainty allows us to remain anchored in light, transforming fear into faith and despair into revelation. **This goes far beyond positive thinking, which can bleed into the category of toxic positivity**. Feel your anger and sadness! Feel your fear! Feel every emotion—the full spectrum. Sit with them, and then create space. Allow certainty to seep in. Certainty connects us to a frequency where healing, miracles, and synchronicities happen. This is why spirituality isn't something we rent for two hours every Sunday—it's a state of being we embody daily.

My father recently passed at the incredible age of 91. I didn't understand his faith when I was young. He spent his life in service, and back then it felt like his devotion pulled him away from us. Now I understand that it was the very thing that allowed him to show up for his family and for the world.

I used to think faith meant constraint. But as discipline creates freedom, faith and spirituality create purpose. It's been repeatedly demonstrated in Blue Zones, those concentrated areas across the globe where centenarians live in higher-than-average numbers, where people who live with meaning recover faster, stay sharper, and experience less depression and anxiety.[17] As we age, we begin to feel the impermanence of material successes. Yet the soul is eternal. Spirituality is the process of remembering a truth in this quote often attributed to French philosopher Pierre Teilhard de Chardin: "We are not human beings having a spiritual experience, but spiritual beings having a human experience." Fear of endings transforms into gratitude for beginnings. Mortality becomes not a punishment, but a passage, a transformation.

I'm more like my dad than I thought. The first thing I do in the morning is pray—before coffee, before I brush my teeth, before I eat anything. Prayer is a nonnegotiable, a sort of cleansing in its own right; a cleansing of the internal. It is setting an intention before the day even begins. Though our modalities differ, my dad and I shared a goal of helping others. Every person has the capacity for spirituality, whether you realize it yet or not. It's the space where your gifts meet someone else's need. You don't need a title to share them; you just need a reason.

That reason is your purpose.

When I look at the five elements as a whole, this one—spirituality—always comes first for a reason. It sets the tone for everything that follows. My morning prayer is followed by meditation and a morning walk with my Pomeranian outside. When asked how I feel on the days I don't pray, meditate, and walk outside, I can't even fathom an answer because the ritual is that much a part of my being. There isn't a morning where I don't pray, meditate, and walk. You can eat clean, move daily, and take your supplements, but if you lack something to believe in, a force higher than you that drives you forward, you'll always feel like something's missing.

Spirituality, believing in something greater than yourself, is that missing piece. It often looks like ordinary life, not congregations, sermons, or pews. With it, even the smallest act becomes sacred, and life itself becomes an evolving expression of divine light. It doesn't require staunch rituals, only rhythms that resonate with who you are and, more importantly, who you're becoming.

# Chapter 5

# Mindset

*Your life will only expand to the size of the beliefs
you're willing to outgrow.
—Carlos Cintron*

Now back to my therapist telling me about my crooked chakras—whatever the hell that meant.

Something about our consultation stuck with me, and I continued going to this guy. One evening, after one of the earlier therapy sessions, I typed *how to learn to meditate* into Google, and what populated the page has changed my life in the years since. I found the research and teachings of Dr. Joe Dispenza:

"Lose your mind and find a new one."

"If you want a new outcome, you will have to break the habit of being yourself, and reinvent a new self."

"If you want a new personal reality, you'll need to change your personality."

It rattled me. And it landed. That evening I bought his meditation course *The Formula* and decided to show up consistently.

At the time, quieting my mind felt like trying to stop a freight train by standing in front of it. My thoughts didn't just happen, they barreled through me, flattening me, and crippling every cell in my body. You see, our thoughts don't happen in a vacuum. They start in the mind and manifest through the body, creating a feeling in accordance with that thought.

Here's an example inspired by Dr. Dispenza's book *Breaking the Habit of Being Yourself*. Say you leave for work in the morning feeling perfectly neutral. You're sitting in your car, half zoning out on the monotonous drive before you suddenly recall a heated discussion you had with a colleague days prior. You replay the conversation, your thoughts launching every clapback you wished you'd said in the moment. Your neck gets hot, your brow furrows, and temples tense. You're angry.

It doesn't take much for something else happening outside of your mind to fuel your anger. Someone cuts over a lane to make their exit right in front of your bumper, snapping you out of your imaginary argument. That's the final straw—expletives are spewed, horns blare. By the time you pull into the office parking lot, you're fuming. And the day hasn't even begun! But it's too late, and your body has succumbed to an emotion, anger, from what started only in your mind—a singular thought! It's more than mental, it's chemical.

Psychologists say the body becomes addicted to the emotions of our thoughts—whether anger, guilt, shame, or stress—much like a drug addict becomes addicted to his vice. He only needs a small amount at first to achieve the high. Eventually, his brain adapts to the poison and starts to feel more normal with it in his system than without, and the dosage becomes larger to accommodate the thinker's tolerance.[18] Rinse and repeat. To break the cycle he has to retrain his brain. Mindfulness techniques affect neurotransmitter systems in the brain. For example, individuals who regularly practice meditation have been found to have higher levels of gamma-aminobutyric acid (GABA), the most common neurotransmitter in our central nervous system. GABA produces a calming effect in the brain and thus, the body. Decreased GABA levels are linked to severe neurological and mental health conditions.[19]

The average person has around 6,000 thoughts a day, and the body listens to every single one.[20] Science can't (yet) detect the nature and content of those thoughts, but you can probably estimate what percentage of your own thoughts are negative and repetitive. Your thoughts aren't passive background noise. They're biological commands. Each one sends an electrical signal through the brain, which triggers a cascade of chemical messengers in the body. Those messengers tell your cells what to do—how to feel, how to behave, and yes, how to age. This is called epigenetics. Your genes play a role, but so does your environment and behavior. The environment you create inside your brain, each thought you entertain (consciously or unconsciously) can turn genes on or off.[21] Ultimately, you're in control.

All of this can sound complex, but here's the point: Your brain isn't fixed, and neither is your biology. Every thought, every choice, every moment you exercise awareness of your internal state is a chance to rewire your operating system.

Think about this. Two people can share the same genetic predisposition to inflammation, anxiety, or disease, but live radically different outcomes based on their mindset and habits. Your biology does not write your biography. It's your response to it that does. That's what Dr. Joe means by "to change your personal reality, you must change your personality." Neuroscientists call this neuroplasticity—the brain's ability to change its structure and function through repetition.[22] You literally rewire yourself with your thoughts. Every time you catch a self-depricating thought or interrupt an old pattern of worry and replace it with acceptance, curiosity or calm, you're creating new neural pathways in your brain. Like strength training for the mind, consistency compounds.

Meditation is the best mindfulness tool for rewiring your mind.[23] As I said, it changed my life. But like strength training, it takes practice. After all, it's called a meditation practice, not a meditation perfect. The word meditation means *to become familiar with*. It refers to becoming familiar with your own mind and its contents—your thoughts and emotions—through mindfulness practices that cultivate awareness and focus. Meditation isn't always occurring in stillness either. There are moving meditations, reclining meditations, mantra meditations (where you repeat words or phrases aloud), breathwork mediations, and visualization meditations to name a few.

The meditations I began with, however, were to be practiced sitting up straight in stillness. At first I couldn't sit one minute before my mind started racing. Dr. Joe explained that we all have an analytical mind and with daily practice the mind and body would eventually acquiesce. **I'd spent years training my body to take on the toxicity in my mind—complain, blame, shame, replay.** So I treated becoming conscious of my unconscious thoughts like reps: five minutes, then ten, then twenty. After two months I found myself meditating for an hour! Sometimes I stood up from a session bawling my eyes out. Not from frustration, but because something chemical was unfolding in my brain and body. I added breathwork to the practice, pulling energy up the spine from my root chakra. When done correctly, spinal fluid touches your pineal gland, your third eye chakra, and creates a magnetic charge, something that can only be described as an orgasm in the brain!

Gradually and without fanfare, things shifted. I experienced this inexplicable happiness. The inflammation dissipated. Rumination subsided. For the first time in a long time I was in control of my mind and my body.

I didn't want the magic to end. I continued to meditate and soon learned visualization. You're probably thinking: *What does this have to do with aging?* Did you know that you can heal and command your body with meditation and visualization? Science calls it coherence: the alignment of your heart, brain, and body into one rhythmic, synchronized state.[24] It's how athletes—Serena Williams, Arnold Schwarzenegger, and Tom Brady for example—were known to practice visualization techniques, mentally rehearsing successful outcomes ahead of big events. When you enter coherence, the nervous system shifts from survival to creation. That's when healing happens.[25] For me, the inflammation faded, my sleep improved, and my energy returned. But more than that, my outlook changed. I began to notice my thoughts before they owned me. I could redirect them. That's when I truly understood what practitioners mean when they say that your body becomes a mirror of your mind. You can literally become what you think about!

I often wonder why more people don't utilize this form of meditation. When done consistently, a pharmacy of feel-good chemicals are released in your body that not even Big Pharma can replicate. I'm sure you've heard the term *mind over matter*, which is exactly how visualization works in the context of meditation. Focus not just on what you want, but how your desired outcome would **feel** *in your body*. Would you feel energetic? Inspired? Relieved? Quiet-minded? What would your breath be doing in the reality of your desired outcome? Is it shallow in your chest or deep and steady down to your belly? Adopt those feelings as though your desire—the BEST case scenario—is happening right now. You will get the outcome. It may not be in five minutes and maybe not even in five years. But when you sharpen your desires to the *feeling* that surrounds it and not the desire itself, it's magic. Dr. Joe asked the question: "If our thoughts can make us sick, then can our thoughts make us well?" As a neuroscientist who repaired his own spine with his mind after a cycling injury that should've left him paralyzed from the waist down, the answer is a resounding yes.

Your mindset about aging works the same way. Tell yourself you're declining, and your biology will oblige. Tell yourself you're adaptable, capable, and curious, and your biology will rally behind that too. In fact, a study from Yale has shown that **people with positive beliefs about aging live, on average, 7.5 years longer** than those with negative ones—even after accounting for gender, socioeconomic status, and health conditions.[26] That's not luck. That's belief influencing biology. When you begin to observe your thoughts instead of identifying with them, when you learn to choose the ones that serve you, you're rehearsing that future into reality.

———————

Most people underestimate the link between mindset and our biology. Your thoughts are not background noise; they form the biological blueprint. I lived that concept decades before I uttered the word neuroplasticity at my first real bodybuilding show, once I had a coach and had been training with precision for my endomorphic body type (more on the three body types in the next chapter). After sixteen weeks of training and prep, the day had finally come.

I was only 33 years old and in the best physical shape of my life up until that point. But I woke up feeling so tired and depleted. Brian Crull assured me that is exactly how I was supposed to look and feel. I had to dig deep and find another gear. I dragged myself out of bed, stepped into the bathroom, flipped on the light, and looked at myself in the mirror. "I am a champion," I told myself. I knew in that moment I had done everything to get myself in peak condition, and I was ready. I was spray tanned (the signature look bodybuilders sport to help the judges see contrast on the muscles) the night before. The only thing left to do was top it off with oil.

When I was finished, I gazed at my reflection and began to cry. My body looked like one of the guys in the magazines I used to idolize. I realized in that moment I felt more myself than I ever had before. At 6 feet tall, 193 lbs, 6% bodyfat, I was showing up to the Southwest Natural stage in peak physical condition. Backstage after my group was finished posing for the judges I was approached by many other bodybuilders and spectators, all congratulating me on my physique and stage performance. I placed second in my category, but I felt like a winner, especially as a natural competitor among the enhanced guys. On that stage among professionals who were all magazine material, I finally felt like I belonged.

That morning, I understood something I couldn't have articulated then: I had already won long before stepping on stage. I had built the body in my mind first. The training was just how I made it real. I had done the work and built inner confidence that would've made my younger self proud. That's all that mattered after the stage lights went dark and the crowd went home.

So if spirituality gives you your *why*, mindset illuminates the *what*. Meditation is the bridge between the two—the *how*.

It's where science meets the soul. Aging stops being fixed and starts becoming mutable…a conversation with your potential and an invisible hand winding your biological clock *backwards*. The further science advances, the more scientists and researchers are seeing science intersect with spirituality.[27]

Mindset is where change starts, but it's not what sees you through to the finish line. You may be able to think your way into good health, but you must back yourself by living it. In the coming pages we'll explore how movement, nutrition, and functional medicine work together to keep your body capable of matching the mindset you're building. Feeling good in your mind is supported by feeling good in your aging body, and when you move for longevity, your body will show you gratitude in its response.

*Chapter 6*

# Movement

*If exercise were a pill, it would be the most
prescribed medicine in the world.*
*—Carlos Cintron*

## Movement is Free Medicine

Working out is my favorite part of my day. It puts me in a great mood and productive frame of mind, and it sets the tone for the whole day. Moving your body builds confidence and self-esteem and makes you look and feel younger! Discovering exercise as a teenager changed the trajectory of my whole life, and it's a routine I've been practicing for almost five decades. Movement is energy in motion, the secret to keeping your mind sharp, your body capable, and your spirit youthful. The human body was designed to move! It's your most powerful and most accessible longevity medicine.

When you make movement a daily ritual you activate every system in the body, release endorphins, balance hormones, and build emotional resilience. Movement isn't optional; it's essential.

## How Much Should You Move?

Most healthy adults should aim for 150 minutes of moderate-intensity aerobic exercise per week.[28] That's only 20 minutes a day! Moderate intensity exercise would be anything like brisk walking, cycling, or swimming. If higher intensity movement is your thing, aim for at least 75 minutes of running, high-intensity interval training, or fast-paced sports per week. For enhanced benefits like weight management, double it to around 300 minutes per week.

Movement happens beyond the gym. Not everyone thrives under fluorescent lights surrounded by weight racks, and that's OK! **Exercise is not defined by location or intensity, but by intention.**

Move anywhere:

- A brisk walk at sunrise
- Cycle through your neighborhood
- Dance in your living room
- Hike in nature
- Paddleboard, kayak, or swim
- Chores done with energy and purpose
- Gardening, martial arts, or yoga in the park

When you move your body with consistency and intentionality, blood circulates, mitochondria awaken, and your body becomes a living expression of health.

## Exercise in the Gym and The Power of Environment

The gym is more than just equipment. It's a sanctuary for transformation. For me, the power of music and rhythmic *clink* of steel, the grunts of effort, and the shared energy of others striving to become stronger, better versions of themselves creates an environment for accountability and inspiration. When you step into a space filled with like-minded people pushing their limits, or perhaps putting one foot in front of the other to push through their day, their energy transfers to you. On days when your drive is low the gym community sustains your momentum.

Training in group environments has been shown to boost motivation levels and positively influence your attitude and emotional response to exercise, turning your workout into a ritual of consistency and connection.[29] The gym doesn't just build muscle, it also builds mental toughness, structure, and self-belief.

When you surround yourself with people who inspire you to grow, whether in the gym or in your community, "motivation" stops being fleeting and turns into *part of who you are*; it becomes discipline.

## Movement and the Brain

**If exercise were a pill, it would be the most prescribed medicine in the world.** It improves mood, memory, energy, and focus, while lowering inflammation and disease risk. When you move, your brain releases a natural pharmacy of chemicals—endorphins, norepinephrine, serotonin, and dopamine—that lift your mood and sharpen your mind.[30] After two traumatic brain injuries, I had lived with irritability, anxiety, and brain fog for years. Back then, I didn't have words for it. I only knew that the gym made me feel better. I didn't need studies to tell me that movement helped me think clearly, sleep better, and handle stress. I could feel it.

Research from the American Psychological Association shows that regular physical activity reduces symptoms of anxiety and depression and strengthens the brain's ability to handle stress.[31] People who move consistently experience less burnout and recover faster from mental fatigue.

Exercise increases blood flow to the brain, improving oxygen delivery and nutrient exchange. It also stimulates neurogenesis, or the creation of new brain cells, especially in the hippocampus, the region responsible for learning and memory.[32] In other words, *movement keeps your brain younger.* Harvard researchers have even found that muscle mass itself is linked to longevity. People with higher muscle mass have lower all-cause mortality rates, regardless of body fat percentage. That means the simple act of maintaining strength—not extreme training, only staying active—directly correlates with living longer.[33]

I didn't know it at the time, but exercise probably saved my life. Decades ago, when I first started lifting a couple of sandweights in my driveway, I wasn't doing it to prevent disease or build longevity. I was doing it to find myself underneath an exterior I felt forced to bear. Looking back, I can see how movement became the first building block in my TBI recovery and the beginning of my journey toward reverse aging.

Movement became a form of therapy. Every rep, every early morning in the gym gave me something that medication never could: control. I was doing so much more than building muscles; I was building trust with a body I'd previously felt betrayed by. I believed it could take care of me as long as I took care of it. But you don't have to be a bodybuilder, or even naturally athletic, to reap the same benefits I did back in my 20s. My training changes every decade, so let's break it down for you to train functionally and intelligently at every age and every stage.

## Movement by the Decades

Each decade of life brings a new rhythm—new goals, priorities, and new ways to train smarter. Longevity is built by training better for your body's evolving needs. I've built a program for you to jumpstart your journey in each decade of life, whether in the gym or anywhere else that inspires you to get moving.

### In your 30s, build the foundation.

You're in your physical prime. This is the decade to establish consistency and build lean muscle mass that will support you for decades ahead.

### Example workout routine:

Strength training 4–5 days/ week, 20 minutes cardio 2–3x/ week (cycling, incline walking, or on the stairclimber)

### Split example:

Monday: Upper Body + 20 minutes cardio
Tuesday: Lower Body

Wednesday: Yoga/recovery walk or full body weight training

Thursday: Upper body + 20 minutes cardio
Friday: Lower body

Saturday: Yoga/recovery walk + 20 minutes cardio

Sunday: Yoga/recovery walk

**Goal:** Build strength and consistency, push yourself hard, and establish metabolic resilience

**In your 40s, maintain your muscle and master balance.**

Your metabolism begins to shift and recovery takes longer. Strength training becomes nonnegotiable—it's your armor against aging and hormonal decline.

**Example workout routine:**
Strength training 4 days/week, add focused core stability exercises. Moderate intensity or circuit-style cardio 3x/week (rowing machine, sled push, air bike)

**Split example:**
Monday: Full-body weight training + cardio

Tuesday: Yoga/recovery walk

Wednesday: Full-body weight training + cardio

Thursday: Yoga/recovery walk

Friday: full-body weight training + cardio

Saturday: Full-body weight training

Sunday: Yoga/recovery walk

**Goal:** Preserve muscle tone, optimize hormones, and support recovery with balanced movement

**In your 50s, move for longevity.**
Joint health, mobility, and posture take center stage. Combine moderate strength training with functional movement and low-impact cardio.

**Example workout routine:**
Full-body circuit training 3–4 days/week plus cardio 3–4x/week (brisk walking, swimming, or elliptical) and core stability movements

**Split example:**
Monday: Full-body weight training

Tuesday: Low-impact cardio (walk outside, swim, elliptical)

Wednesday: Yoga/Pilates class

Thursday: Full-body weight training + low-impact cardio (walk outside, swim, elliptical)

Friday: Low-impact cardio (walk outside, swim, elliptical)

Saturday: Full-body weight training

Sunday: Recovery walk and stretch/yoga

**Goal:** Maintain bone density, muscle mass, and flexibility

**In your 60s, focus on mobility, stability, and mindfulness.**

Flexibility, balance, and stability become key. Keep strength movements controlled and intentional. Prioritize injury prevention, recovery, and joint care.

**Example workout routine:**
Lighter weight training 3 days/week , 4–5 days/week cardio (walk, water aerobics, stationary bike, or dance-based fitness)

**Split example:**
Monday: Full-body light strength training

Tuesday: Low-impact cardio (walk outside, swim, bike, dance)

Wednesday: Low-impact cardio (walk outside, swim, bike, dance)

Thursday: Full-body light strength training

Friday: Low-impact cardio (walk outside, swim, bike, dance)

Saturday: Full-body light strength training

Sunday: Yoga/Pilates class + low-impact cardio (walk outside, swim, bike, dance)

**Goal:** Maintain joint mobility, coordination, and muscle to prevent falls early

**In your 70s, movement is medicine.**
Movement now becomes a form of self-care and soul nourishment. Every step is an investment in independence and vitality.

**Example workout routine:**

Gentle full-body, low-impact weight training 2–3 days a week, cardio 5 days/week (walking, incline walking, yoga, chair yoga, tai chi, water movement)

**Split example:**

Monday: Yoga class

Tuesday: Full-body, low-impact weight training

Wednesday: Yoga class

Thursday: Incline walk

Friday: Full-body, low-impact weight training

Saturday: Zumba class

Sunday: Recovery yoga or rest

**Goal:** Support balance, mobility, and longevity through gentle consistency

**Remember to check with a health care professional before starting a new exercise program, especially if you have any concerns about your fitness or haven't exercised for a long time. Also check with a health care professional if you have chronic health problems, such as heart disease, diabetes, or arthritis.**

## You Don't Stop Moving Because You Age—You Age Because You Stop Moving.

In medicine, memory loss, specifically Alzheimer's, is considered type 3 diabetes or diabetes of the brain.[34] My mother doesn't remember that my father has passed. Too often she relives the grief as if it just happened. Watching her move through that confusion has been one of the hardest things I've experienced in my life. Dementia is something I wouldn't wish on my worst enemy—that disconnection from everything that makes life full and meaningful.

Dementia develops through insulin resistance, inflammation, and reduced blood flow—the same issues that lead to diabetes and heart disease.[35] Watching my mom decline while working in regenerative medicine was a gut punch, startling me awake unlike any lab discovery or medical journal ever could. I realized something so simple and yet profound: **Movement isn't optional. It is medicine.** It supports cognitive function just as much as muscular strength.

## What Happens When You Stop Moving?

Over 53% of US adults don't meet the Centers for Disease Control and Prevention (CDC) physical activity guidelines for aerobic exercise. **Lack of movement is one of the biggest risk factors for nearly every chronic disease.**[36]

According to the Department of Health and Human Services, roughly half of American adults—about 117 million people—live with at least one preventable chronic disease. Regular physical activity can positively influence seven out of the ten most common: heart disease, diabetes, obesity, certain cancers, high blood pressure, stroke, and depression.[37]

The problem gets worse with age. As we get older:

- Nutrient absorption declines, making deficiencies in essential micronutrients like vitamin D, B12, magnesium, and zinc more common.[38]

- The body becomes less efficient at using protein, which makes maintaining muscle harder.[39]
- The microbiome shifts, impacting immunity, cognition, and inflammation.[40]

Sarcopenia—the gradual loss of muscle mass and strength—starts as early as your 30s if you don't actively counter it. It affects about 5% to 13% of people ages 60 to 70, and up to 50% of people who are 80 or older. The result is slower metabolism, loss of balance, more falls, and even faster cognitive decline.[41]

**Making Movement a Habit**

I used to think motivation was the key to consistency. It's not. The secret is discipline in routine, or *automaticity*. The University College of London conducted a study that shows it takes 66 days to build a habit.[42] James Clear, author of *Atomic Habits*, wrote an article explaining why the findings are not disheartening but inspiring, in comparison to the widely accepted belief that it takes only twenty-one days to form a habit. He highlights how embracing longer timelines helps us realize that habits are a process, not a singular event.[43]

You can't rely on feeling inspired every day. You need structure that makes movement automatic. That's where training changed everything for me. When I was prepping for my bodybuilding competitions, I didn't have the luxury of waiting until I "felt like it." I trained because it was on the game plan and part of the process. The discipline I built through competition prep became the lasting reward and much more valuable than where I ended up on the podium. You don't need to be perfect; you need to show up. Each time you do, you're teaching your brain and body to trust each other again. Movement is free medicine and the thread that connects physical health, cognitive health, emotional stability, and spiritual vitality. It keeps your body young, your hormones balanced, your brain sharp, and your energy magnetic.

Whether you lift weights or lift your grandchildren, train in the gym or dance under the stars, movement is how you honor life itself and the body you've been given. But the movement must be fueled with *real* nutrition. The food readily available to us, even those labeled organic, don't pack the same nutrients they once did.[44] In the next chapter, you'll learn *how to stay fueled and nourished for life.*

# Chapter 7

# Nutrition

*Let food be thy medicine and medicine be thy food.*
*—Hippocrates*

## Eat Like You Want to Be Here in 50 Years

As a certified health and wellness coach, bodybuilder, and someone who lived with obesity until my mid-teens, this fourth element is dear to my heart. I attribute my overall well-being to nutrition because it is the number one factor that contributes to disease and mortality. It also affects your emotional state, your confidence, and your self-esteem. When nutrition is neglected you're susceptible to depression and emotional eating—a dangerous combination that works against your health and longevity.

If movement is medicine, food is the pharmacy.

## Most of Us Are Undernourished, Not Underfed

We live in a culture that gets food wrong, counting calories instead of nutrients. We obsess over macros, trends, and willpower, but we forget the simple fact that food is information for your cells. Every bite you take is a message to your body saying "heal" or "harm." You won't outtrain, outthink, or outsupplement a poor diet.

Up until the age of 23, I ate like most people trying to lose fat and gain muscle mass: smaller portions, more protein, carbs and fats in moderation. When I began studying the *Encyclopedia of Modern Bodybuilding*, I started to understand how the results I was trying to achieve in the gym came from the kitchen. Nutrition provides the building blocks for muscle growth and recovery while exercise provides the stimulus for that growth. It also taught me this key fact: not all bodies are the same. Arnold teaches that everyone falls into **three main body types**. Some of us are a combination of the three. I switched my approach to be guided more by this science than blindly restricting cravings or borrowing someone else's meal plan that may work well for their body. But their body wasn't my body.

## Understanding Your Body: The Three Somatotypes

Each body has its own rhythm and design. Aligning your nutritional strategy, fasting routine, and lifestyle habits with your somatotype is an effective way to optimize body composition (your body's proportions of fat, muscle, water), regulate metabolism, and reverse biological aging.[45]

Humans are metabolically diverse. Our skeletal frame, hormonal profile, and muscle-to-fat ratio all influence how we metabolize nutrients. The somatotype system—*ectomorph, mesomorph,* and *endomorph*—provides a foundational map for nutrient distribution, portion control, and metabolic efficiency.[46]

Let's break down each body type with a guide for how to fuel with food. This is the same guide that, with the help of my coach and rigorous training, got me into single-digit bodyfat percentage for competition purposes. **I do not recommend losing body fat below teen digits. I was following professional bodybuilding requirements and protocols. Consult your healthcare professional before beginning any new nutrition regimen.**

### Ectomorph

- Traits: Naturally slim, light and lean frame, fast metabolism, struggles to gain muscle or weight, burns carbs quickly, often prone to low blood sugar or fatigue if meals are skipped
- Goal: Build lean muscle and strength without overtraining, while stabilizing blood sugar and hormone balance
- Ideal macronutrient split:
  » **Protein:** 25–30%
  » **Carbohydrates:** 50–55%
  » **Fats:** 20–25%

**Meal frequency:** 5–6 balanced meals per day or 3 main + 2 snacks (eating every 3–4 hours)

**Recommended foods:**
- **Proteins:** chicken breast, eggs, wild salmon, turkey, Greek yogurt, whey isolate protein powder (if tolerated)

- **Carbohydrates:** oats, brown rice, quinoa, whole grains, yams, bananas, berries
- **Fats:** avocado, almond butter, olive oil, chia seeds, nuts

**Portion guide** (per meal):

- 1 palm-size of protein
- 2 cupped hands of complex carbohydrates
- 1 thumb of healthy fats

**Additional tips:**

- Use liquid calories (smoothies and shakes) to meet caloric goals
- Drinking a protein shake within 30 minutes following a workout improves glycogen restoration, ensuring muscles have adequate fuel to repair and grow
- Limit cardio; focus on *compound weight/resistance training* 3–4x/week

**Mesomorph**

- Traits: Naturally athletic, symmetrical build with balanced muscle mass, gains muscle and loses fat easily
- Goal: Maintains lean muscle mass while fine-tuning fat levels and hormonal balance
- Ideal macronutrient split
  - » **Protein:** 30–35%
  - » **Carbohydrates:** 40–45%
  - » **Fats:** 20–25%

**Meal frequency:** 4–5 meals per day with balanced macros

**Recommended foods:**

- **Proteins:** chicken, lean beef, wild caught fish, eggs, tempeh
- **Carbohydrates:** sweet potatoes, quinoa, fruit, vegetables, brown rice
- **Fats:** olive oil, walnuts, coconut oil, flaxseed

**Portion guide** (per meal):

- 1 palm-sized portion of protein
- 1 cupped handful of carbs
- 1 thumb of healthy fat

**Additional tips:**

- **Moderate resistance training** and 2–3 high-intensity interval sessions weekly for best results
- **Adjust carbohydrates** around workouts; reduce on rest days
- Focus on **nutrient timing**—carbohydrates post-workout, fats earlier in the day

**Endomorph**

- Traits: Rounder frame, higher body fat percentage, stronger appetite, powerful strength potential, slower metabolism, higher insulin sensitivity challenges
- Goal: Maintain lean muscle mass, enhance fat metabolism, improve insulin sensitivity
- Ideal Macronutrient Split
  - » **Protein:** 35–40%
  - » **Carbohydrates:** 20–25%

» **Fats:** 35–40%

**Meal frequency:** 3 main meals + optional small protein-based snack; *intermittent fasting can be highly beneficial, but consult your physician before trying*

**Recommended foods:**
- **Proteins:** white fish, chicken, turkey, egg whites, low-fat Greek yogurt
- **Carbohydrates:** veggies, berries, quinoa, legumes
- **Fats:** avocado, nuts, MCT oil, olive oil, fatty fish

**Portion Guide** (per meal):

- 1.5 palms protein
- ½ cupped hand carbs
- 1.5 thumbs healthy fats

**Additional tips:**
- Carbohydrates are best consumed post-exercise
- Avoid high-glycemic foods, like white bread, white potatoes, corn, white sugar
- Resistance and metabolic circuit training 4–5x/week will control fat and preserve lean muscle

*Don't forget vegetables! Fiber-rich and cruciferous greens like spinach, broccoli, kale, cauliflower, and asparagus are good for every somatotype.*

I'm an endomorph: naturally stockier, prone to storing fat easily. Once I started eating for *my* body type—higher protein, moderate complex carbs, low sugar, and timing macronutrients more precisely around my training—it was game on. I leaned out, had more energy, and for the first time felt like nutrition was working in support of my body instead of against it. It wasn't anything fancy; I prioritized whole foods and consistency, adopting a 70/30 approach.

Something else that helped me, and I'm sure could help other recovering emotional eaters, is learning about the *gut-brain connection*. The *vagus nerve*, located in the brainstem on either side of your neck, travels down the neck and enters the chest cavity and abdomen, where it branches out to connect the gut to the brain.[47] It takes approximately *15-20 minutes for your brain to register fullness after eating.*[48] You can foster a stronger connection between your brain and stomach by eating slowly and presently. Avoid scrolling on your phone and watching television. Swap it for listening to background music or simply enjoying the company of those around you. The Japanese practice of *Hara hachi bu* is a **reminder to stop eating at 80% full to prevent overeating.**[49] Another helpful trick is to put your utensils down between every few bites to stay conscious during the act of eating. A gut-brain imbalance affects neurotransmitter production; 95% of serotonin is produced in the gut![50]

I realized nutrition isn't about perfection at all, but about patterns. What you do *most of the time* is what shapes your body and biology. Food is your most direct avenue to influencing how you age.[51]

## Fasting, Inflammation, and Autophagy

Autophagy or "self-eating", is a process where the body clears out old, dysfunctional cells. Intermittent fasting ignites autophagy, which is beneficial for inflammation because it decreases inflammatory markers as the body resets itself.[52] Intermittent fasting recycles misfolded proteins, reducing neurodegenerative risk when it's made part of your routine.[53] Extra support for organs involved in autophagy can be achieved through supplementation, which we'll cover in depth in the next chapter.

Autophagy ages you backwards. It promotes new collagen and fibroblast (connective tissue) regeneration, improving skin elasticity, and giving skin that bouncy, hydrated, and youthful quality.

What counts as a "fast"? Intermittent fasting to reach autophagy is defined by controlled cycles of eating and abstaining designed to optimize metabolism, insulin sensitivity, and cellular repair. Here are some common intermittent fast protocols. Water and herbal tea (no caffeine) are allowed and encouraged during fasting periods. *Hydration is key!*

| Type: | Fasting hours: | Eating window: | Best for: |
| --- | --- | --- | --- |
| 12:12 | 8pm–8am | 8pm–8am | beginners, hormone balancing |
| 16:8 | 8pm–12pm | 12pm–8pm | fat loss, mental clarity |

| 18:6 | 7pm–1pm | 1pm–7pm | advanced cellular repair |
| --- | --- | --- | --- |
| 24 hr (2x/ week max) | 8pm–8pm | N/A | deep detox, autophagy boost |

Not all fasts are created equal and not every individual is a good match for every fasting window. I follow a 16:8 hour fast, and a 48-hour fast bi-monthly. Recommended frequency for those with stable blood sugar is to follow a 16:8 fast 4–6 days per week for maintenance. Once a week, you may introduce one 24 hour fast for deep cellular renewal. **Consult your health care professional before beginning a new fasting regimen.**

## The Biology of Food Addiction

Stress leads to spikes in cortisol, causing you to crave sugary and fatty foods. *Emotional eating* activates our dopamine pathways, similar to how narcotics do. Victims of food addiction find themselves in a crash-and-crave cycle that derails insulin and serotonin. Chronic emotional eating paves the way for chronic inflammation, which can result in obesity, metabolic, and mood disorders.[54]

We're all susceptible to emotional eating, but you don't need to fall victim to it. Identify your triggers, whether it be boredom, stress, loneliness, or something else.

Here's how you can start combatting emotional eating starting today.

1.  **Pause** and breathe before you begin eating, asking yourself if you're *really* hungry, or if your brain is tricking you.

2.  **Hydrate**, hydrate, hydrate! Dehydration mimics hunger cues.

3.  **Disrupt and replace** the ritual. Start by giving yourself grace and compassion (because we can't shame ourselves into healthier habits) and instead go on a short walk, dance around for a few minutes, throw yourself into a task you've been putting off, or journal and meditate.

4.  When you're ready to return to the table, **choose whole foods** to stabilize your blood sugar and reduce cravings.

## The Food System Problem

Here's another layer to the story. Even when we *do* eat well, our food isn't what it used to be. Industrial farming and Big Agriculture have changed how we grow food—and not for the better. Monocropping, pesticides, and rapid harvesting have stripped our soil of nutrients. The consequence of these practices means produce available to us contains *20–40% fewer vitamins and minerals* than it did fifty years ago.[55] Factor in long shipping times, storage, and processing, and by the time our vegetables reach our plates they've lost much of their original nutrition. Same for animal products—livestock fed on corn and soy instead of fats have lower omega-3s and more inflammatory fats that we ingest by proxy.[56] This may feel overwhelming, especially given we're no longer hunter-gatherers who know the source of all our food. The control is out of our hands. But we can't become apathetic. Let this remind us that food alone often isn't enough anymore. We'll talk about supplements in the next chapter, but for now this is the takeaway: *nutrient density matters more than calorie count.*

**Food addiction is an epidemic.** Modern processed foods are designed for addiction. Chronic exposure to packaged food, fast foods, pizza, chocolate, ice cream, chips, and sugary drinks desensitize the brain to normal food rewards, intensifying cravings. Making processed foods a staple in your diet causes chronic metabolic dysfunction and inflammation. *Rewire the reward system.*[57] Transition to *whole foods* and gradually reduce processed sugar, instead enjoying natural sugars from fruits, maple syrup without additives, and organic local honey. Watch your cravings for processed foods reduce and disappear like magic! By increasing protein and whole sources of omega-3 fatty acids you can regulate your dopamine naturally. Take back control; you have other options than to be at the mercy of the processed food epidemic.

## Play the Long Game

Eating one salad doesn't make you healthy, just like one skipped workout doesn't make you unfit. Eat mostly whole foods, stay hydrated, and manage your blood sugar most days, and your body compounds those benefits over time. Each day you eat in alignment with your goals, you're making a deposit. Every day you don't, you're making a withdrawal. One can't break you, but a pattern of ultra-processed eating will. The goal isn't to eat clean 100% of the time. It's to eat clean *most* of the time so your body can work with those resources to heal and perform when you need it.

Make changes in baby steps: one better breakfast, one less soda, one more home-cooked meal, and shop the perimeter of your grocery store. Small improvements stacked daily add up faster than you think. You don't have to crack the code to your ideal meal plan or track every macro to age well. You just have to eat like you want to be here in 50 years.

Filling the Gap Between Food and Nutrition with Functional Medicine

In America alone:

- 65% of people are vitamin D deficient,

- 40% are low in magnesium, 80% fall short on omega-3 fatty acids

- An astounding 90% aren't meeting minimum requirements for at least one essential nutrient.[58]

These deficiencies are *essential* vitamins for cell function. Vitamin D influences over 200 genes. Magnesium regulates more than 300 enzyme reactions. Omega-3s lower inflammation and support cognitive health. Supplements reinforce and fill those gaps, but they're not without their own drawbacks. When you think of food as medicine, supplements are how you ensure the medicine works. But when *anyone* can develop and sell a supplement, quality control goes down. Fillers, gums, artificial flavorings—everything that causes an inflammation response in your body—spreads on shelves around the world. Which brings us to the final puzzle piece in reversing your biological age: RVRSBL Wellness and functional medicine.

# Chapter 8

# Functional Medicine

*A healthy person has a thousand wishes,*
*a sick person just one.*
*–Confucius*

When something feels off, you can accept the first answer you're given or you can listen to your intuition and ask one more question. Most people stop after the first. Functional medicine begins after the second.

Can you recall a time you waited weeks, or maybe months, for an appointment with your doctor or a specialist; spent time meticulously tracking and compiling a list of symptoms and questions; and sat in a waiting room for 45 minutes only to be brought back and have 10 minutes with your doctor? This isn't your doctor's fault; it goes way above them to the systemic problem of Western medicine and Big Pharma. Have you left those appointments feeling more confused and alone and, ultimately, worse than when you came in? I understand. It's time you take back control of your health. I never want you to leave another doctor's office feeling defeated again.

Traditional medicine looks for disease, not dysfunction, managing symptoms over systemic cause. Functional medicine asks different questions: Why is this happening? What's exacerbating it? Where are the patterns, and how do we stop them from repeating?

Preventative regenerative medicine is the opposite of conformity. It's curiosity, made clinical.

I started having heart palpitations a few years ago around age 60. Nothing major at first, just a flutter here and there. But as the days went on it got noticeably worse. I was thinking, *What's going on? I'm in great shape, and I take care of myself…*

I made an appointment with my doctor, who ran an EKG and told me I had an arrhythmia. His next sentence was a surprise. "I'm going to refer you to a heart specialist." My gut sank. I'd worked hard for decades to eat well, lift and live clean, age well; and now I was being told something was wrong with my heart. The doctor also told me that my bloodwork suggested anemia.

"Are you taking iron?" he asked.

I wasn't. I'd recently cut back on red meat and thought a general multivitamin was enough to make up the difference. He didn't recommend dietary changes or further testing. I took the heart specialist referral and left the visit without any real answers. That night I went home and did what curiosity always drives me to do—I researched. I found studies linking mild anemia and vitamin B deficiencies to heart palpitations and fatigue. I learned that being "within the normal range" doesn't mean "optimal." Traditional doctors only test for the range. Functional medicine pinpoints an individual's optimum and then creates a plan to get them there. The next day, I started supplementing with liquid B6 and B9 and added an iron formula plus vitamin C to help with absorption.

Three months later the palpitations were gone.

If I'd gone to the heart specialist they would've prescribed something to suppress the arrhythmia and more than likely introduce a few new symptoms. Instead, I treated the cause. That experience reinforced how I thought about medicine forever.

## The Problem With "Normal"

My least favorite words to hear when I'm sick or feeling less than my best are "everything looks normal."

Conventional labs test to see if you're sick. Functional medicine tests to see if you're *thriving*.

The problem with normal is when you get bloodwork done results are compared to population averages as the "normal range." But those numbers come from a sample of the general population, and the general population isn't very healthy. Normal just means common. And, if you recall from chapter one, *not* accepting what's common as normal is the byproduct of the inner work you've been doing.

Functional medicine looks at optimal ranges for *you*. Where energy, organs, cognition, digestion, and hormones perform at their best in your body. For example: Your iron might not be technically low, but if it's suboptimal for your metabolism you'll feel the symptoms long before it ever flags on a standard panel. That's what happened to me. I wasn't sick and my heart wasn't in trouble; I was underperforming. And the body always whispers before it screams. The foundation of The 5 Elements of Life is learning how to tune in *and* tune out so you're able to recognize your body's whispers.

## What Functional Medicine Actually Is

Functional medicine is an advanced approach that looks at the entire human ecosystem. It connects your genes, microbiome, hormones, nutrition, environment, and mindset. Instead of asking "What drug fixes this symptom?" it asks "What imbalance(s) caused this in the first place?" Functional medicine gives you a more complete picture. Pioneered by Dr. Jeffrey Bland in the 1990s, functional medicine emerged as a scientific evolution of a more personalized approach to medicine. His work has created The Institute for Functional Medicine (IFM), where biochemistry, genomics, and nutrition are integrated into modern clinical practice.[59]

Six in ten US adults have at least one chronic disease. Four in ten have two or more. And 86% of our healthcare spending goes to managing those conditions, not preventing them.[60] We're living in a reactive system that's keeping us sick, not a proactive one that's aiding our healthspan. Functional medicine flips that model. It asks us to participate in our health journey instead of outsourcing it.

## Two Sides of the Longevity Spectrum: Preventative and Regenerative Medicine

### Preventative Medicine: The Practice of Staying Well

**Preventative medicine (PM) focuses on reducing risk factors before disease develops**—aka Elements of Life numbers 1–4! Core principles of PM are detection of predispositions through genetic markers, identification of inflammation dysfunction *before* symptoms appear, and using functional labs to track *healthspan metrics* beyond only disease. There's a theory that genetic testing is going to be part of the intake process when you go to a new doctor in the not-so-far future. The first piece of information gathered as a new patient will be genetic tests to provide the blueprint for your body and what you need. Everybody's different, and genetics don't lie. PM will make standard pinpointing genetic deficiencies and recommending proper supplements, peptides, and therapies customized for you.

Genetic (fixed) and epigenetic (mutable) tests reveal predispositions toward inflammation, cognitive decline, or poor detoxification. Blood panels measure nutrient absorption and hormone balance. From there, your plan is tailored to *you*.

Brad Mullins, the founder of DNA Regimen where I became an ambassador, first brought genetic testing into my view. I experienced how eye-opening the knowledge of my parents' genetic histories could be for my health. Not so much for longevity, because they were in their 80s at the time. I wanted to find out if the gene for Alzheimer's and dementia showed up, so I ordered a kit online to be shipped to my house. One simple mouth swab and a few weeks later, a geneticist called to read my results and send the full report to my primary care physician. That blueprint removed the guesswork, giving me a chance to mitigate disease and catch any markers early.

## When Should You Start?

Start now! Prevention begins before dysfunction. The earlier you begin optimizing mitochondrial health, hormone balance, and detox pathways, the slower your biological clock ticks.

------

## Regenerative Medicine: The Science of Reversing Decline

**Regenerative medicine (RM)** is the science of restoring and repairing what's been damaged by age, disease, or injury. It teaches the body to remember what healing looks like, like a map it can follow. Core principles of RM include activating *autophagy* for cellular turnover and repair; regenerating damaged tissue and strengthening cell communication; restoring *mitochondrial* and *hormonal function*; and reversing *inflammation-driven degenerative* changes. So that all sounds advanced and sciency. How do we tell the body where and how to heal?

**Our bodies are expert healers** under the right conditions. Each cut that closes and each bruise that fades is proof the map for healing already exists inside us. RM is like GPS that helps healing efforts find the fastest route. RM research is not new. It's been happening for years and continues to develop, and not only in industry labs and clinics. Traditionally trained physicians are adopting more RM practices into their clinics around the world.

There are three main levels of regeneration:

- **Molecular:** repairs DNA and cell membranes damaged by oxidative stress
- **Cellular:** replaces or rejuvenates cells that have stopped functioning properly
- **Tissue:** regenerates whole structures like cartilage, bone, or skin

Tools used to achieve all levels of regeneration include **peptide therapies, exosome therapy, mitochondrial support,** and **bioregulators** that upregulate gene expression and tissue repair.

## When Should You Start?

A smart time to begin RM is in your 40s when early degeneration and hormonal shifts begin. RM is also increasingly being used preventatively to optimize specific health functions such as digestion, energy production, and overall cellular health even in the 30s, especially for high-performance individuals.

For example, a patient in their 30s with genetic markers in detoxification and methylation pathways may begin with preventative nutraceuticals and peptide support. By the 40s and 50s regenerative peptides and bioregulators are layered in to reverse decline and continue decreasing biological age.

## Founding RVRSBL, and RVRSBL GeneCode

### RVRSBL: Time to Turn Back Time

Along my functional health journey as a lab representative, I discovered a problem: the wellness industry was saturated with one-size-fits-all supplements. Most companies were pushing products that helped their bottom line rather than gave consumers true solutions. That's why I developed RVRSBL and RVRSBL GeneCode.

In 2020, during one of the most uncertain times in history, I found clarity. The world was forced to slow down and in that stillness I was met with the space to start asking better questions. *What if we could reverse our biological age instead of just masking symptoms of aging?* I had spent years in the beauty and wellness industry helping people look better on the outside, but walking around as living proof of how real transformation must start within. During COVID, a glaring weakness in the medical field was revealed in the reactionary nature of the system. Patients came out of 2020 looking for new, preventative ways to take care of their health after the wake-up call that was the pandemic. Whether you're for or against the vaccines, everyone experienced fear to some degree. We launched a holistic approach to preventative medicine. RVRSBL GeneCode tests and identifies 123 genetic markers across nine different health categories essential for longevity.

By utilizing the science that drives RVRSBL GeneCode, people would have their genetic blueprint in hand. But what's next? How does one address any deficiencies?

The supplements I saw on shelves lacked science. I was aware of the aging population statistic shared at the beginning of this book, but in case you'd like a reminder—by 2030, 1 in 6 people will be aged 60 or over.[61] I knew I wanted to come out with longevity products. But many people are needle-phobic and administering at home isn't accessible. Could I find a way to develop an oral peptide with the same benefits?

The lab I was involved with had created a patented delivery system that allows oral peptides to pass the gastric acid in the stomach, meaning they don't dissolve before getting absorbed. I first decided to focus only on these oral peptides with the lab and make them the most effective, well-researched, and bioavailable supplements on the market. It was of utmost importance that I had reputable partners behind the initiative, so utilizing the inroads I had made was a no-brainer.

I wanted to create more than a supplement brand—I was out to spur a longevity movement where people received not just a product, but access to education and tools for living better longer.

It was important to me as a TBI survivor that *our* formulations were developed to cross the blood-brain barrier. That protective membrane keeps toxins out, but also keeps a lot of the key ingredients in a supplement from ever reaching the brain, which defeats the purpose of a supplement. By formulating them to cross the blood-brain barrier, RVRSBL's products are more bioavailable, especially for people with traumatic brain injuries where communication between neurons can be disrupted.

We use fat-soluble delivery systems so nutrients don't pass through your digestive system and dissolve in stomach acid; they make it to the cells that need them.

Functional medicine starts with questions. When you join RVRSBL, you take a personalized health quiz to identify everything from age and body type to how inflammation could be manifesting—those whispers and signals your body is sending asking for more support. Based on the results we provide *stacks*, a multi-level approach rather than a single approach to a single symptom. Because everything is connected: Your gut affects your brain. Your sleep affects your hormones. Your stress affects your digestion. Internal wellness creates external beauty. Our products focus on internal wellness first before building your stack with products that focus on the external.

## The RVRSBL Trinity™: Peptides, Nutraceuticals, and Bioregulator Stacks

Say you get your genetic testing done, you have your results in hand, and you walk into a supplement shop ready to stock up on the support *your body* specifically needs. Not only are you overwhelmed at walls and walls of options, but your cart quickly fills up with dozens of products. You're wondering how much this is going to cost each month and how you're going to schedule taking dozens of supplements throughout your busy days. RVRSBL solves this problem by targeting three categories to combine products specially developed to work together for your longevity: **peptides, bioregulators, and nutraceuticals**. These supplement groupings are specially designed to work together for total bio-optimization without draining your energy or your pockets. The key to any new health routine is *simplicity*—and we've spent five years developing a simple way to build a personalized bio-optimization regimen without compromising quality.

## Peptides

Peptides are amino acids that signal repair in the body, and as we age those peptides diminish dramatically, and we begin to experience more symptoms. Support from oral peptides relieves a slew of those symptoms and addresses autoimmune, cognition, hormonal imbalances, weight loss…the list goes on, but that'd be a whole other book!

One of the most well-studied uses of peptide therapy is in the treatment of **chronic pain**, making it a popular treatment among athletes, as well as fitness enthusiasts and anyone seeking improved overall health and wellness. It's also been applied to **autoimmune disorders,** like rheumatoid arthritis and multiple sclerosis. Peptides have been shown to increase insulin sensitivity and reduce appetite, making them a potential treatment option for diabetes and prediabetes.

## Bioregulators

Bioregulators are peptides too, but smaller—two to four amino acids compared to peptides' four to fifty. Bioregulators can bind themselves to a cell and penetrate the cell wall and cross the blood-brain barrier, making them incredible short-chain amino acids for regenerating organs. Both forms of oral peptides have the advantage of working on the body long-term when taken daily, whereas injectables work at a higher level but for a shorter amount of time.

## Nutraceuticals

Nutraceuticals, *nutrition + pharmaceuticals*, are targeted natural compounds found in food and other natural sources that act on molecular pathways to improve function and longevity. Unlike standard supplements that simply "add" nutrients, nutraceuticals activate biological pathways that encourage healing, repair, and prevention. They support *homeostasis*—the body's ability to maintain internal balance—while optimizing organ function. With the rise of genetic testing and biomarker analysis, nutraceuticals are prescribed based on an individual's unique biology. This precision approach allows targeted support, personalized at the cellular level.

## The FDA, Big Pharma, and the Future

The FDA views RM / Cell therapies as drugs, not supplements. It's important to add cell therapies because nutraceuticals, oral peptides, and bioregulators are not considered cell therapies, and it's what I will be offering on my RVRSBL platform/marketplace.

Big Pharma doesn't make money on prevention. There's little incentive to promote therapies that help people need fewer prescriptions. That's why it's on us—the practitioners, the patients, the curious—to keep asking questions and seeking out reliable, ethical providers.

This feels mainstream to those familiar with the research or any athlete or celebrity wealthy enough to take advantage of these therapies on a more regular basis. But it's not the first line of defense the general population's minds turn to when they're seeking medical support. That's all going to change; regenerative medicine is not "the future." It's already here.

---

I still receive regenerative treatments once a year as part of my antiaging protocol. For the rest of the year I rely on the same foundation I've built this entire book on—spirituality and mindset, movement, nutrition, and targeted supplementation. My daily RVRSBL stack of peptides, bioregulators, and nutraceuticals wouldn't be even half as effective without the lifestyle. But with the therapies in play, I'm able to more easily maintain a good lifestyle. One doesn't happen without the other.

# Chapter 9

# The Choice Is Yours

The answers to the uncertainties you've carried about getting older have always been within you. Release what no longer serves you. You *can* live differently, and you already are!

I'm here at 62 planning the next 50 years of my life. That's my mindset.

My journey was one to save myself. I only realize this looking back. The exercise routine I cemented as a teen, supplements I began taking in my 20s, and habits built and enforced over decades of consistency mitigated what could've been more severe TBI symptoms. The full-circle moment of that journey is this book—my mission to help a billion people. I want to touch the world and leave it better than I found it, like my father did. And this isn't the destination, it's only the beginning. RVRSBL Ingestible Beauty & Wellness is a love letter to my past self. I developed a pattern of returning to the research when faced with a challenge. And the research is solid—spirituality, mindset, movement, nutrition, and functional medicine will allow you to squeeze every ounce of vitality out of your mid-to-late years.

Every nourishing meal, quality night's sleep, walk in nature, and moment of laughter and connection are investments in your future vitality. Like compound interest, their benefits multiply with consistency over time. Start later and you can still make progress. But start early, and you build resilience that will carry you through life's inevitable storms. You create a foundation Western medicine alone cannot offer. With this model, you're more than merely existing. You're truly living.

Personal growth isn't a phase; it's a lifelong practice. The goalposts are constantly moving because each time you expand your comfort zone a new goal comes into view. I work on myself every day and I always will because the greatest project you'll ever work on is *you*. So don't underestimate your human potential. Don't listen to the noise that says you're getting old. Don't conform—evolve. Believe in yourself, because no one is coming to save you. Your transformation is your responsibility.

## Living The 5 Elements of Life

I live **The 5 Elements of Life** every day because they've become my foundation for longevity, clarity, and peace. You don't have to be perfect when you start. What matters is that you begin at all, and that you follow this framework in order.

Each morning, wake up and **connect with your higher power;** give gratitude for the miracle of being alive.

**Sit in stillness**—even one minute of imperfect meditation can change your day. Don't reach for your phone; come back to your breath as a home base and soak in the present.

**Move your body**—walk, train, stretch, dance! Because movement is medicine.

**Fuel your body with real food,** not processed poison, and hydrate like your cells depend on it, because they do.

And finally, **optimize your system**: take your supplements, ask questions, get your comprehensive genetic bloodwork done, and invest in your healthspan as much as your lifespan.

Master these five elements and you'll discover what it truly means to live with purpose.

Most people forget how to believe in themselves and in reinvention. Living unconscious and in the past, repeating the same story, lamenting about how they *used to be*. That phrase is a toxic self-fulfilling prophecy of decline. To every *used to be*, I ask: What have you done lately? At 62 I started salsa lessons, launched a new company, and wrote this book—not because I had to, but because I refuse to live small. If you want to live life to the fullest you must step out of your comfort zone and challenge yourself; that's what keeps you young at heart and keeps the old at bay. The moment you slow down, you signal to your subconscious that it's over and your cells obey that command. Stop that behavior. Instead, reprogram your mind through visualization: close your eyes, breathe deeply, play meditative music, and *see* yourself young, vibrant, strong, unstoppable. After five or ten minutes, open your eyes…you've just met the next version of you. *Because you don't age by years; you age by mindset. And you become what you think about.*

Every morning, you wake up to face the same battle—you vs. you.

One version of you wants to grow, evolve, and take charge of your life.

The other wants to stay comfortable, to play it safe, to cling to the illusion of security.

And when it comes to health, most people choose safety—not because they can't change, but because they've fallen victim to the status quo. We live in a world obsessed with instant gratification, where everyone is searching for a magic pill that doesn't exist. What does exist is a choice. That choice is a conscious decision to take responsibility for our lives, our health, and our futures.

That choice is what's waiting for you after the final page.

When you align yourself with The 5 Elements of Life, everything changes. But you must commit. Not partially. Not occasionally. Fully. The framework you've taken the time to learn here isn't a call to perfection, it's a checklist. If you're solid on one or two elements already, great! Focus your efforts on one you haven't yet mastered. Don't skip an element and don't expect overnight miracles. Do them consistently, and you will experience transformation beyond what you thought possible.

Life is amazing. The proof is in the doing; if you do it right you're not fading. Muscle maturity, wisdom, and every beautiful milestone that comes with aging is a gift—one to look forward to.

My prayer for you is simple: realize that it's always *you vs. you*. The power has been and always will be within you. Make the choice to change with joy, with faith, and with inspiration.

When you do, life doesn't only get better—it becomes extraordinary.

I dedicate this chapter to all the readers who came this far and are determined to act!

*Time To Turn Back Time.*

With love and gratitude,

Carlos

# About the Author

Carlos Cintron is a regenerative and preventative medicine expert and lifelong student of human potential. With more than four decades of experience in fitness, nutrition, and transformation, Carlos blends cutting-edge science with lived wisdom to challenge the conventional narrative around aging.

His philosophy was shaped early in life. At four years old, Carlos suffered a traumatic brain injury. Instead of limiting him, it ignited his commitment to understanding the body's ability to heal, adapt, and regenerate. Growing up as an overweight, struggling kid, Carlos learned firsthand how environment, belief, and behavior shape biology. Those early battles became the foundation of his calling: to help people rewrite the stories their bodies have been carrying for years.

After decades as an award-winning creative director in the beauty industry, Carlos made a radical choice—to turn his focus inward and transform his own biology. His career was built at the intersection of regenerative medicine, epigenetics, functional wellness, and mindset, drawing from thousands of clinical conversations and years of collaboration with leading physicians, researchers, and innovators.

A former all-natural bodybuilder, Carlos approaches longevity through a holistic lens—one that honors spirituality, mindset, movement, and nutrition as the true drivers of healthspan. His work is rooted in the belief that *internal wellness creates external beauty,* and that the human body is far more capable than most people have been taught.

Carlos founded RVRSBL, and RVRSBL Genecode, a longevity company inspired by his years overcoming injury, chronic inflammation, and metabolic dysfunction. RVRSBL's mission is simple: provide holistic, science-backed solutions that support the body's innate ability to repair and thrive. His work reflects a single, powerful promise: You can turn back time from the inside out. www.rvrsbl.com.

Today, Carlos uses his platform to inspire people of every age to reclaim their vitality and redefine what it means to age. He now lives in New York City, where he begins each morning walking through Central Park with his spirited Pomeranian—a simple daily reminder that movement, joy, and connection are medicine for a long and meaningful life.

When he's not working or speaking about wellness and longevity, you'll find Carlos in the gym, reading, or spending time with his daughter Sophia—always learning, always curious, always evolving.

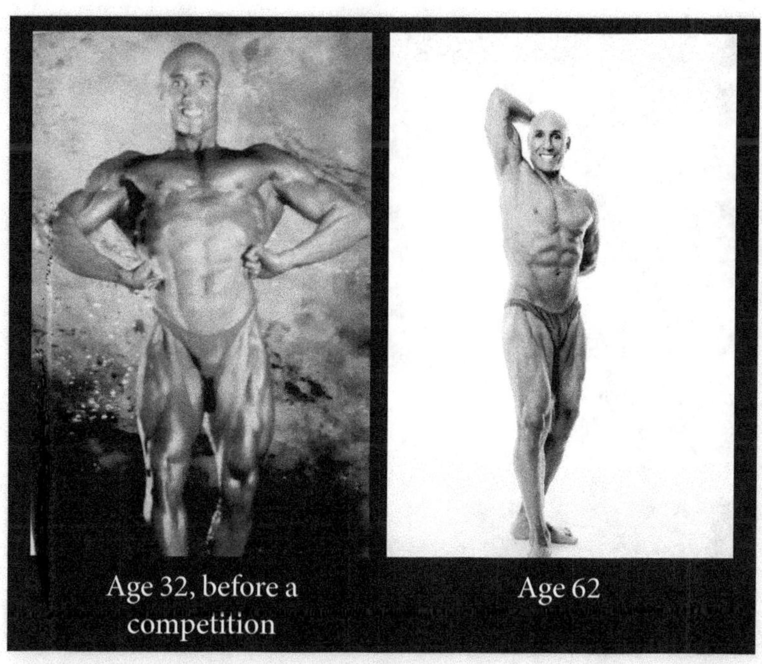

Age 32, before a competition

Age 62

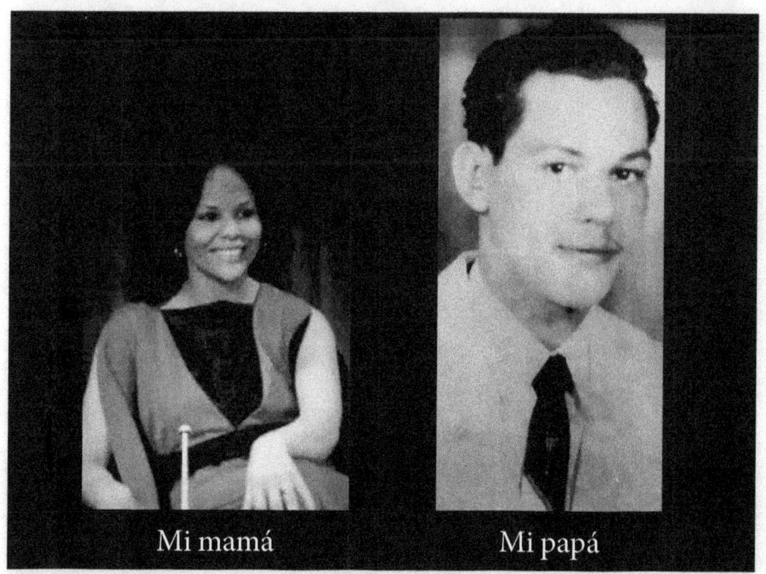

Mi mamá

Mi papá

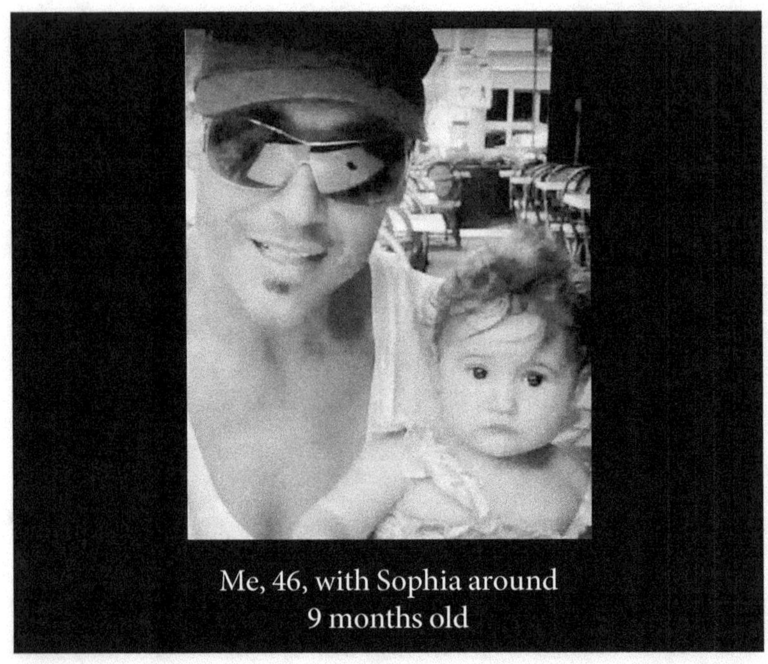

Me, 46, with Sophia around
9 months old

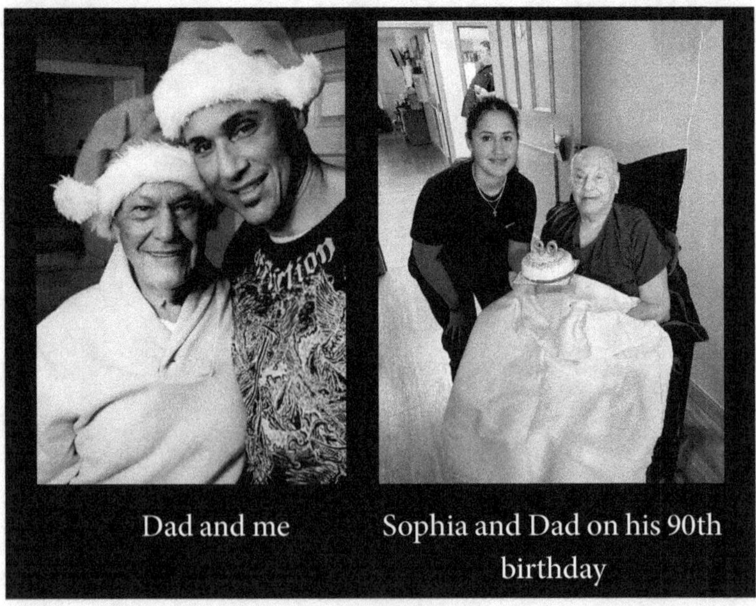

Dad and me

Sophia and Dad on his 90th
birthday

# Notes

1. World Health Organization, "Ageing and Health," Knowledge Action Portal on Noncommunicable Diseases, accessed July 31, 2025, https://www.knowledge-action-portal.com/en/content/ageing-and-health.

2. Abby Smith, "Mayo Clinic Q and A: Lifespan vs. Healthspan," Mayo Clinic News Network, September 14, 2024, https://newsnetwork.mayoclinic.org/discussion/mayo-clinic-q-and-a-lifespan-vs-healthspan/.

3. Michiko Sakaki, Ayano Yagi, and Kou Murayama, "Curiosity in Old Age: A Possible Key to Achieving Adaptive Aging," Neuroscience & Biobehavioral Reviews 94 (2018): 343–362, https://doi.org/10.1016/j.neubiorev.2018.03.007.

4. Eden A. Getahun and Katie L. Sevier, "Dr. Jeffrey D. Rediger's Pillars of Spontaneous Healing," Harvard Crimson Magazine, March 10, 2022, https://www.thecrimson.com/article/2022/3/10/rediger-spontaneous-healing/.

5. Lulu Xie et al., "Sleep Drives Metabolite Clearance from the Adult Brain," Science 342, no. 6156 (2013): 373–377, https://doi.org/10.1126/science.1241224.

6. T. Wilmanski, C. Diener, M. Rappaport, et al., "Gut Microbiome Pattern Reflects Healthy Ageing and Predicts Survival in Humans," Nature Metabolism 3 (2021): 274–286, https://doi.org/10.1038/s42255-021-00348-0.

7. Office of Research on Women's Health, "Autoimmune Diseases and Women," National Institutes of Health, last modified April 24, 2025, https://orwh.od.nih.gov/OADR-ORWH.

8. Ibid.

9. World Health Organization, "Mental Health," fact sheet, October 8, 2025, https://www.who.int/news-room/fact-sheets/detail/mental-health.

10. Healthy Minds Network, The State of Student Mental Health 2023–2024: National Report (September 2024), https://healthymindsnetwork.org/wp-content/uploads/2024/09/HMS_national_report_090924.pdf.

11. American Heart Association, "More than Half of US Adults Don't Know Heart Disease Is Leading Cause of Death Despite 100-Year Reign," January 24, 2024, https://newsroom.heart.org/news/more-than-half-of-u-s-adults-dont-know-heart-disease-is-leading-cause-of-death-despite-100-year-reign.

12. Sonya Collins, "2024—First Year the US Expects More than 2M New Cases of Cancer," American Cancer Society, January 17, 2024, https://www.cancer.org/research/acs-research-news/facts-and-figures-2024.html.

13. José Ostaiza-Cardenas et al., "Epigenetic Modulation by Life-Style: Advances in Diet, Exercise, and Mindfulness for Disease Prevention and Health Optimization," Frontiers in Nutrition 12 (2025): 12408607, https://doi.org/10.3389/fnut.2025.12408607.

14. Claudio Franceschi and Judith Campisi, "Chronic Inflammation (Inflammaging) and Its Potential Contribution to Age-Associated Diseases," Journals of Gerontology: Series A 69, suppl. 1 (2014): S4–S9, https://doi.org/10.1093/gerona/glu057.

15. Donald G. Phinney and Mark F. Pittenger, "Concise Review: MSC-Derived Exosomes for Cell-Free Therapy," *Stem Cells* 35, no. 4 (2017): 851–858, https://doi.org/10.1002/stem.2575.

16. Claudio Franceschi and Judith Campisi, "Chronic Inflammation (Inflammaging) and Its Potential Contribution to Age-Associated Diseases," Journals of Gerontology: Series A 69, suppl. 1 (2014): S4–S9, https://doi.org/10.1093/gerona/glu057.

17. Roundtable on Population Health Improvement, Lessons from the Blue Zones®, in Business Engagement in Building Healthy Communities: Workshop Summary (Washington, DC: National Academies Press, 2015), https://www.ncbi.nlm.nih.gov/books/NBK298903/.

18. Lee Daniel Hawker-Lecesne, "What Is Emotional Addiction? Understanding the Definition and Effects," The Cabin Chiang Mai, April 26, 2025, https://www.thecabinchiangmai.com/blog/emotional-addiction/.

19. Andrea Calderone et al., "Neurobiological Changes Induced by Mindfulness and Meditation: A Systematic Review," Biomedicines 12, no. 11 (2024): 2613, https://doi.org/10.3390/biomedicines12112613.

20. Robby Berman, "New Study Suggests We Have 6,200 Thoughts Every Day," Big Think, April 19, 2022, https://bigthink.com/neuropsych/how-many-thoughts-per-day/.

21. Ostaiza-Cardenas et al., "Epigenetic Modulation by Life-Style."

22. Matt Puderbaugh, "Neuroplasticity," StatPearls [Internet] (Treasure Island, FL: StatPearls Publishing, May 1, 2023), https://www.ncbi.nlm.nih.gov/books/NBK557811/.

23. Calderone et al., "Neurobiological Changes Induced by Mindfulness and Meditation."

24. "Coherence Healing: A Path to Achieving Balance and Well-Being," Quantum Clinic, April 15, 2025, https://www.quantumclinic.com/blog/coherence-healing-a-path-to-achieving-balance-and-well-being/524.

25. Ibid.

26. Jane E. Dee, "Becca Levy and the Fight against Ageism," Yale School of Public Health, May 5, 2023, https://ysph.yale.edu/about-school-of-public-health/communications-public-relations/publications/public-health-magazine/article/becca-levy-and-the-fight-against-ageism/.

27. Mashiyat Ahmed, "Spirituality and Science Can Be Two Sides of the Same Coin," The Varsity, February 5, 2024, https://thevarsity.ca/2024/02/05/spirituality-and-science-can-be-two-sides-of-the-same-coin/.

28. ODPHP Staff, "Current Guidelines," Office of Disease Prevention and Health Promotion, 2024, https://odphp.health.gov/our-work/nutrition-physical-activity/physical-activity-guidelines/current-guidelines.

29. L. Alison Phillips and Jacob Meyer, "Group Exercise May Be Even Better for You than Solo Workouts—Here's Why," Department of Kinesiology and Health, Iowa State University, October 16, 2024, https://kin.hs.iastate.edu/group-exercise-may-be-even-better-for-you-than-solo-workouts-heres-why/.

30. Kristen Weir, "The Exercise Effect," Monitor on Psychology 42, no. 11 (December 2011), https://www.apa.org/monitor/2011/12/exercise.

31. Ibid.

32. Lindsay Warner, "A Guide to Combatting Sarcopenia and Preserving Muscle Mass as You Get Older," Harvard Health, September 6, 2024, https://www.health.harvard.edu/staying-healthy/a-guide-to-combatting-sarcopenia-and-preserving-muscle-mass-as-you-get-older.

33. Ibid.

34. Suzanne M. de la Monte and Jack R. Wands, "Alzheimer's Disease Is Type 3 Diabetes—Evidence Reviewed," Journal of Diabetes Science and Technology 2, no. 6 (2008): 1101–1113, https://doi.org/10.1177/19322968 0800200619.

35. de la Monte and Wands, "Alzheimer's Disease Is Type 3 Diabetes."

36. Centers for Disease Control and Prevention, "FASTSTATS – Exercise or Physical Activity," December 10, 2024, https://www.cdc.gov/ nchs/fastats/exercise.htm.

37. Franceschi and Campisi, "Chronic Inflammation (Inflammaging)."

38. Centers for Disease Control and Prevention, "About Chronic Diseases," October 4, 2024, https://www.cdc.gov/chronic-disease/about/ index.html.

39. Varsha D. Badal et al., "The Gut Microbiome, Aging, and Longevity: A Systematic Review," Nutrients 12, no. 12 (2020): 3759, https://doi. org/10.3390/nu12123759.

40. Badal et al., "Gut Microbiome, Aging, and Longevity."

41. Warner, "Guide to Combatting Sarcopenia."

42. Philippa Lally, "How Long Does It Take to Form a Habit?," UCL News, September 17, 2009, https://www.ucl.ac.uk/news/2009/aug/how-long-does-it-take-form-habit.

43. James Clear, "How Long Does It Actually Take to Form a New Habit? (Backed by Science)," February 4, 2020, https://jamesclear.com/ new-habit.

44. Muhammad Atiq ur Rehman et al., "Declining Nutrient Composition of Food Crops and Its Impact on Human Health," Frontiers in Nutrition 10 (2023): 1210077, https://doi.org/10.3389/ fnut.2023.1210077.

45. Andrew Payne, "How to Train and Diet for Your Body Type," National Academy of Sports Medicine, accessed September 11, 2025, https://www.nasm.org/resource-center/blog/body-types-how-to-train-diet-for-your-body-type.

46. Ibid.

47. Ibid.

48. Badal et al., "Gut Microbiome, Aging, and Longevity."

49. Jaclyn Tolentino, "A Functional Medicine Doctor Breaks Down Mindful Eating—Without the Wellness Fluff," The Good Trade, October 2, 2025, https://www.thegoodtrade.com/features/what-is-mindful-eating/.

50. Roundtable on Population Health Improvement, "Lessons from the Blue Zones®," in Business Engagement in Building Healthy Communities: Workshop Summary (Washington, DC: National Academies Press, 2015).

51. Jeremy Appleton, "The Gut-Brain Axis: Influence of Microbiota on Mood and Mental Health," Integrative Medicine (Encinitas) 17, no. 4 (2018): 28–32, https://pmc.ncbi.nlm.nih.gov/articles/PMC6469458/.

52. Ostaiza-Cardenas et al., "Epigenetic Modulation by Life-Style."

53. Eirini Lionaki, Maria Markaki, and Nektarios Tavernarakis, "Autophagy and Ageing: Insights from Invertebrate Model Organisms," Ageing Research Reviews 11, no. 2 (2012): 273–282, https://doi.org/10.1016/j.arr.2011.11.001.

54. Hawker-Lecesne, "What Is Emotional Addiction."

55. Rehman et al., "Declining Nutrient Composition of Food Crops."

56. Rehman et al., "Declining Nutrient Composition of Food Crops."

57. Erica M. LaFata et al., "Ultra-Processed Food Addiction: A Research Update," Nutrients 16, no. 6 (2024): 867, https://doi.org/10.3390/nu16060867.

58. Carroll A. Reider et al., "Inadequacy of Immune Health Nutrients: Intakes in US Adults, the 2005–2016 NHANES," Nutrients 12, no. 6 (2020): 1735, https://doi.org/10.3390/nu12061735.

59. Institute for Functional Medicine, "Educator: Jeffrey Bland, PhD," accessed November 20, 2025, https://www.ifm.org/educator/jeffrey-bland.

60. Centers for Disease Control and Prevention, "About Chronic Diseases," October 4, 2024, https://www.cdc.gov/chronic-disease/about/index.html.

61. World Health Organization, "Ageing and Health," Knowledge Action Portal on Noncommunicable Diseases, accessed July 31, 2025, https://www.knowledge-action-portal.com/en/content/ageing-and-health.